W9-BHA-432

THE BIG LITTLE BOOK OF pilates

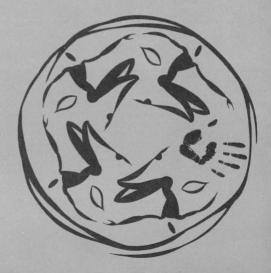

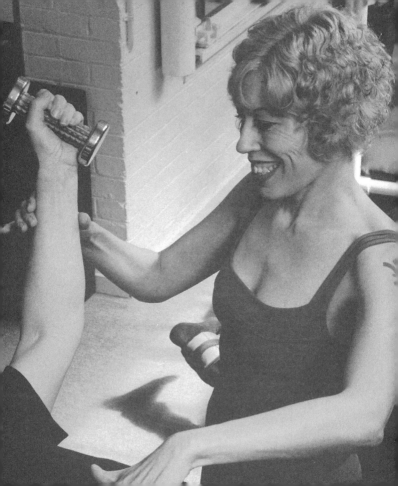

THE BIG LITTLE BOOK OF **pilates**

The only book you'll
ever need

LESLEY ACKLAND

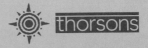

Thorsons
An Imprint of HarperCollins*Publishers*
77–85 Fulham Palace Road,
Hammersmith,
London W6 8JB

The website address is: www.thorsonselement.com

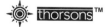

and *Thorsons* are trademarks of
HarperCollins*Publishers* Limited

Published by Thorsons 2003

Text derived from *10-Minute Pilates, 10-Step Pilates,
Pilates Body Power*, and *Pilates with a Ball*

10 9 8 7 6 5 4 3 2 1

A catalogue record for this book is
available from the British Library

ISBN 0 00 717062 9

Printed and bound by Imago

contents

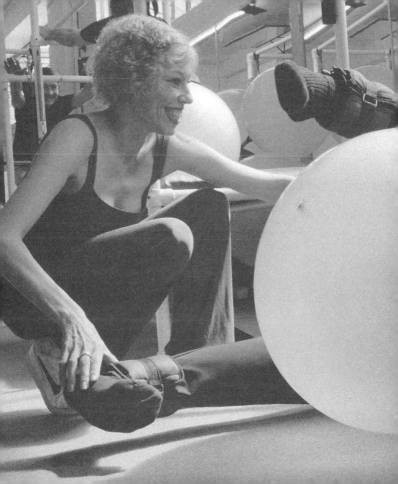

Do you dream of a flat stomach, a longer, leaner body, and superb posture? Do you wish to improve your overall appearance? If so, then Pilates will help you achieve all this – and more. In this book you will discover a unique bodywork system that will help you transform your body and develop a physical presence and energy that exude total confidence and grace.

how to use this book

If you want to become healthier, stronger, leaner, and more supple, my Pilates-based Body Maintenance techniques are designed to work for all ages and all levels of fitness. There are also exercises for pregnancy and specific remedial techniques you can try if you suffer from medical conditions such as a bad back, scoliosis, repetitive strain injury (carpal tunnel syndrome), or sciatica.

While most people have heard of Pilates, few know exactly what it entails. Pilates is a very disciplined, focused form of exercise, designed to strengthen ligaments and joints, increase flexibility, and lengthen the muscles. The main emphasis is on "elongating" the body to create a longer, leaner, and taller silhouette. However, Pilates differs from other exercise regimes by going beyond the purely physical. This is a holistic discipline that integrates the mind, body, and spirit. It is a philosophy of movement that brings about mental and physical integration.

If you have never tried this type of exercise before, you will be surprised by its apparent simplicity. The slow, controlled movements enable energy to move more freely throughout the body. The visualization techniques gently help to focus the mind so that each exercise is executed with ultimate precision. With these exercises there is no need for overexertion. The emphasis is on quality, not quantity. It's not about how much you do but, rather, how you do it. This is good news indeed for those of you who have become disillusioned and bored with fitness programs that may not suit you.

If you want to have a long, lean look, with a minimum of effort in the safest way, you merely have to follow the guidelines in this book. Most of the techniques are based on the idea of using your own body to create resistance, so there is no need for special equipment – unless of course you're going to do the Physio Ball program. The most important thing you need is a willing body and a curious mind. Before you attempt any of the exercises, though, it is important that you first become acquainted with the underlying principles so do read the early chapters first.

In the Introduction I outline the origins of Pilates, and how I have evolved and updated this classic regime to make it more contemporary and accessible. Chapter 1 explains how much easier it is to bring about physical changes when you learn to focus your mind and practice visualization techniques as well.

Chapter 2 covers the basic principles of Body Maintenance, such as the importance of proper breathing, alignment, and movement control. It introduces the key terms that are used throughout the book, and explains the physiological effects of Body Maintenance techniques on your body. For

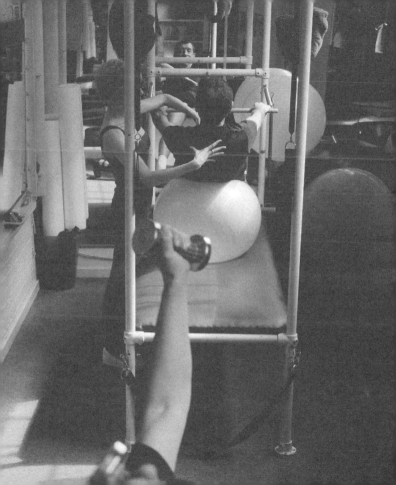

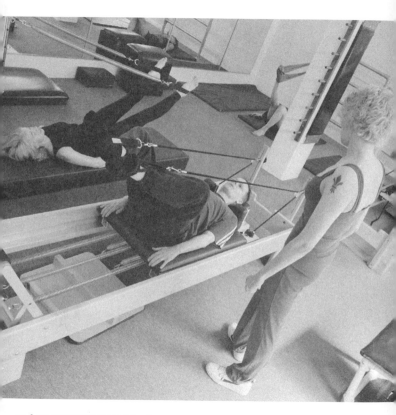

practical advice on clothes, safety, equipment, and how to do the programs, turn to Chapter 3.

The core exercise program is outlined in Chapter 4. Here, you will find all the different types of exercise you can do, at home, every day. They include exercises to tone and strengthen your abdominal muscles, the muscles in your back, your upper body (arms, chest, and shoulders) and your lower body (legs, hips, and thighs), as well as a series of all the essential stretches. Chapter 5 should be of special value to those with a hectic schedule. It features some specific programs that will enable you to squeeze some Pilates into your daily routine – no matter how busy you are. If you suffer from a bad back, scoliosis, repetitive strain injury (carpal tunnel syndrome), or sciatica, you will find the relevant remedial exercises in Chapter 6.

Chapter 7 introduces the Physio Ball and features a routine that anyone can do at home. Physio Balls have become incredibly popular and are particularly appropriate for Pilates exercises. As well as being great for everyday use they have also proved very useful for Pilates-based pregnancy exercises, hence a pregnancy routine using the ball is also included.

The Big Little Book of Pilates promises no quick fixes or sudden improvements. However, with concentration and commitment, the end result will be rewarding and nothing short of enhanced physical and mental wellbeing.

By practicing the exercises in this book I believe that you can achieve the body you want in a controlled, progressive, and intelligent way. Pilates doesn't build bulk, but strengthens weak muscles and stretches tight ones. You can concentrate on one part of the body without straining another.

introduction

Pilates differs from other forms of exercise because it initially focuses on posture. Good posture is essential in realigning the body, which can have you looking and feeling taller, slimmer, and well toned.

The beauty of Pilates is that it is suitable for people of all ages. Notwithstanding your level of fitness, you have the potential for achieving a supple body and reaching a level of "wellness" that you will want to maintain. You should feel good about yourself, which involves an intelligent dialog between your body and mind. Imagery and visualization are very appropriate tools – if you can focus on how you wish to look, the body will most assuredly cooperate. How you picture yourself is reflected in your body language which, in turn, is observed by the world at large. When that language is fluent and flowing you will be aware of it – others will comment on how well you look.

Many people do not have a positive body self-image. Women, specifically, have a tendency to retreat from their bodies as they get older. Pilates can help you achieve the body that you want, and are comfortable with, not the body someone else has judged to be more acceptable. Too often we are held hostage to figures in glossy magazines,

imagining them to be preferable and easily attainable.
I find this unrealistic, even dangerous. We should
acknowledge and appreciate our own bodies and work with
what we are naturally given. Many people do not even
consider the highly desirable aspects of themselves. In
this "media-friendly" generation we are almost
brainwashed into acknowledging "the perfect body" hype,
which is, in fact, merely the fashion of the moment. This
can result in feelings of dissatisfaction and depression.
We have the ability to transform ourselves, to reduce our
self-imposed limitations and tap into our potential – using
my techniques on a daily basis will stretch both the mind
and the body.

Very few of us are born with an anatomically perfect body.
Through habitual misuse, which begins when we are quite
young and continues until we feel discomfort, we can
seriously damage parts of the body. Unknowingly, certain
areas are accentuated and, as we get older, it is more than
likely that one side of the spine will be visibly
overdeveloped. This is when problems manifest
themselves. My Pilates-based exercise program attempts
to create the best body that is possible for you, on your
frame, with the understanding that there is no such thing
as the perfect body. All of us have imbalances. The trouble
begins when an imbalance turns into a physical problem.

For those who have repetitive strain injury (carpal tunnel
syndrome), scoliosis or myriad other problems, Pilates is a

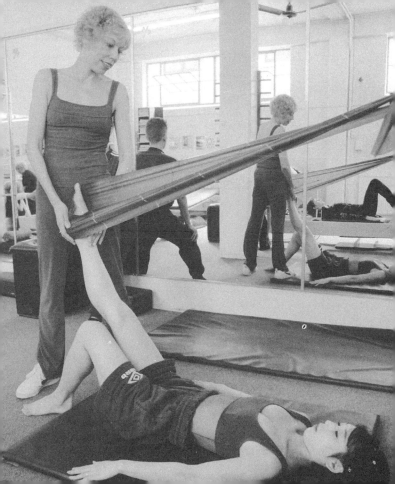

superb tool to use as you begin the journey towards helping and even reversing your condition. I believe that everyone can and will improve and even overcome their physical liabilities, with a safe and gentle group of exercises. You will be amazed at the body's ability to respond and

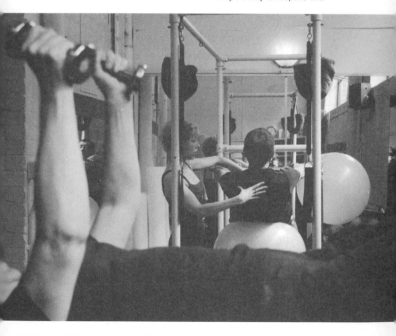

rejuvenate given the correct impetus. For those of you with serious postural problems involving balance, these exercises can change not only your body, but the perception of vulnerability you feel and transmit to others. You will regain your confidence and not live in fear of falling, stumbling, and giving the impression of vulnerability to others who could cause you injury.

I have never met anyone I could not help with my Body Maintenance system. As you begin the following exercises be patient but determined, and feel the body working towards what you have always envisioned – the elegance of a swan's neck, the supple back of a ballet dancer. Feel yourself floating, soaring as you go through your movements. Concentrate on the moment; eventually all will be remembered as you progress. Even those of you who are extremely unfit can look forward to the day you can look in the mirror and not recognize your former selves.

THE ORIGINS OF CLASSIC PILATES

The original concept of Pilates was the brainchild of a German, Joseph Hubertus Pilates. He was extremely frail and weak as a child, but was determined to regain good health. This was the start of a lifelong obsession with fitness and body building, and as a young man he excelled as a diver, skier, and professional gymnast. At the age of 32 he moved to England, where he made a living as a boxer, circus performer, and self-defense instructor.

When the First World War broke out, his career was temporarily cut short. As a German, Pilates was interned in England for the duration of the war. He used this time, however, as an opportunity to re-think and develop his approach to fitness. The result was the first blueprint for a whole new regime, Pilates, which drew upon all the various disciplines with which he was involved. His basic philosophy concluded that the only way to achieve true fitness was through the integration of mind and body. Hence, all his techniques were based on a combination of physical and mental conditioning.

When Joseph Pilates created his unique system of exercise during the early part of the twentieth century, the life style was, in many respects, healthier for the public at large. Without the profusion of cars and mass transportation, walking was not merely a preferred form of exercise but, rather, the most efficient way of getting from place to place.

Many of the injuries and disabilities of today are, in fact, caused by our very modern, machine-oriented society. Repetitive movements on computers and sitting in an office chair for the greater part of the day contradict the physiological needs of the human body. There are also, of course, factors beyond our control, such as genetic traits and unfortunate injuries, which must also be addressed. I knew that I had to expand and enhance the basic principles of Pilates.

BODY MAINTENANCE

Almost 90 years after Pilates was created, physical ailments have changed, but pain has not. Contemporary stress has induced a variety of debilitating afflictions. In 1980 I began developing Body Maintenance, a balanced system of exercise, body shaping, and toning combined with mental improvement and nutrition, based on Pilates. I initially studied with Alan Herdman, who first brought Pilates to the UK. Then I began traveling regularly to New York City to study Pilates there. During my instruction I became aware of a new wave of research on the human body, and I found myself looking at the way physiotherapists were working, particularly at the New York City Ballet, with Physio Balls and Dynabands. I had also become aware of other forms of bodywork, including Feldenkreis and the Alexander Technique.

With Pilates as the main base, I began to integrate methods from a wide variety of sources, including remedial massage, osteopathy, and injury clinics, and created my own unique system of bodywork, which I call Body Maintenance. Over the years, in my own studio at Pineapple Dance Studios in London's Covent Garden, I have worked successfully with people who have suffered from a variety of modern infirmities: repetitive strain injury (carpal tunnel syndrome), chronic back pain (some of which stems from spinal surgery), HIV-related problems, aerobic sprains, extreme obesity, even low self-esteem.

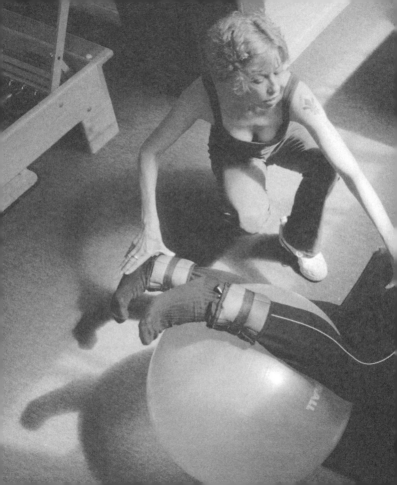

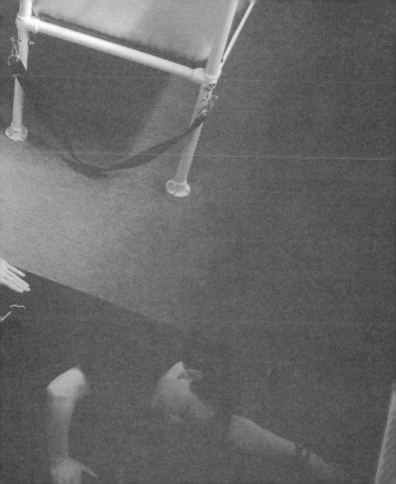

Often called "yoga with machines," the Pilates-based exercises in my studio can incorporate ropes, springs, and pulleys. However, the most important and long-lasting work takes place on the floor. Mat exercises, essential to body mobility and endurance, target weak, under-utilized muscles in the abdomen, lower back, arms, and legs. Based on mat work, the exercises in this book are straightforward, concentrated movements that don't require any special equipment – though of course you can opt for the Physio Ball program. What they do require are a few minutes – in the morning, during lunch, or in the evening. We do have the ability to transform ourselves – using these techniques in a daily routine will stretch both your body and your mind.

For those of you who wish to enhance or change some aspect of your bodies, this routine is simple and straightforward. People tend to use their big muscles for everything. I work on strengthening the smaller muscles, which can give you the shape that you want. You can tone your stomach, thighs, and arms and reshape your buttocks as well. Get into swimsuit shape – look and feel longer, leaner, and more glamorous. There is no limit to what you can expect to achieve. My workout will have you feeling supple, slender, and self-assured. Your entire view of yourself, both physically and emotionally, will improve and you will reach that summit of "wellness" where the mind–body–spirit positively connect. The rest is up to you.

the basics

The main principle of Body Maintenance is that exercise is essentially a mind–body technique. Therefore, when you exercise you should mentally focus on the muscle groups that you are using. Body Maintenance recognizes that it is only through the synchronizing of thought and action that an exercise is truly effective. In order to create a healthy and fit body you need to integrate the mental, physical, and spiritual spheres.

the mind–body connection

MIND OVER MATTER

It has long been established that the mind has an enormous influence on the health of the body. Research shows that the mind has an infinite capacity to induce positive physiological effects, which have both an internal and external effect. You may have noticed that when you're in a good mood you automatically seem to look and feel better. Scientists ascribe this phenomenon to the activity of the billions of nerve cells in our brain, which transmit chemical messages to the rest of the body. Our thoughts and emotions play a vital role in influencing this intercellular communication.

Think for a moment how you feel when you are stressed. Not very pleasant. This is because your body produces an excess of "stress" chemicals (e.g. adrenaline and cortisol) that cause your whole system to speed up. Your heart beats faster, your blood pressure goes up, your breathing becomes rapid and shallow. At times, this type of response is necessary. It is what motivates you when you are faced with a crisis. In large doses this type of reaction can, however, be extremely harmful and lead to all sorts of unpleasant symptoms such as dizziness, shaking, profuse sweating, insomnia, and migraines. It is easy to see what effect negative, stress-inducing emotions can have.

Positive feelings of calm and contentment have a much more beneficial effect, as they induce the body to produce health-enhancing, feel-good chemicals (e.g. endorphins and serotonin) that are vital for wellbeing. They promote a sense of serenity – you breathe more easily and deeply, your heart rate is slower, and your blood pressure lowers. The more relaxed you feel, the less tension you hold in the muscles throughout your body. This has a beneficial effect on your general bearing and posture. Tight, tense muscles make your body shrink and constrict. This stops the energy from flowing freely throughout the body and, in time, this will be reflected in a weak, misshapen musculature.

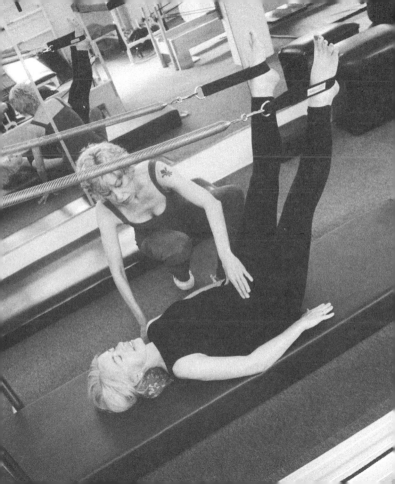

MINDFUL EXERCISE

If thoughts are so powerful, it makes sense to try and harness your thinking to bring about positive changes in your body. This is, in fact, the very essence of Body Maintenance. By learning to execute each exercise correctly you are also allowing your mind to exert a greater influence over your body. With Body Maintenance you only do a limited number of repetitions. You do them slowly, so that you can concentrate more clearly on directing your energy towards what it is that you are trying to achieve. If you view your body in a negative way you will need to reverse your direction of thought. Positive thoughts bring about positive changes.

To ensure that an exercise is of real benefit and will bring about the changes that you desire – for example a strong, straight back – it is necessary to complement each physical action with a mental focus. By practicing creative visualization regularly, you will gradually develop the intellectual and emotional ability to internalize the physical changes you wish to make. Once you've done this, the external changes will start to appear.

As you become aware of your body and its needs, you can consciously start to make changes through exercise. Body Maintenance is based on lengthening and stretching the body to its full potential. This eventually creates a longer, leaner shape, increased flexibility, and a suppleness that promotes a greater ease of movement. These exercises concentrate on strengthening weak muscles and stretching those that are too tight and constricted. What you really want is a body in which strength and flexibility complement each other.

It is possible to totally restructure the way you are. It is not, however, just a matter of getting your body to make the right moves. An integral part of Body Maintenance is the way you perceive the exercise. This is why attitude and creative imagery are so important. Each time you work through a series of movements it is essential that you can envision what it is that you wish to achieve. Painting a picture in your mind helps your body to respond in the right way. This not only makes the whole process more stimulating but also makes the effect of each exercise much more powerful. Initially it may take a while to fully understand the mechanisms. I always tell a new client to expect to do only about 30 percent of what he or she will eventually be capable of doing. It takes about 10 sessions to really comprehend the technique. Body Maintenance is one of the few forms of exercise that gets progressively more difficult, but the results are worth it. In time you will look taller, slimmer, and more toned.

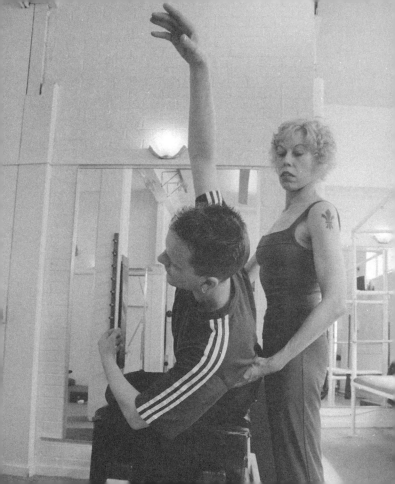

CREATIVE VISUALIZATION

Whatever we create in our lives begins as a basic image in
our minds. Many of these images are unconscious.
Through creative visualization it is possible to alter these
thoughts and pictures. With Body Maintenance, the idea is
to create an image in your mind that will help you to focus
on the area of the body that you are working. This requires
a very deep level of concentration, which does become
easier with practice. On a superficial level, many of the
exercises appear quite simple. How you physically position
your arms and legs, however, is only part of the process.
Body Maintenance, unlike many other disciplines, is
actually much more complex, as with each movement you
must be constantly aware of what your entire body is doing.
You don't concentrate only on the stomach, or the inner
thigh, and exclude the rest of your body. Even when you are
doing a series of movements specifically designed to work
a certain group of muscles, such as your abdominals or
your quads, you must always remember to be equally
focused on the rest of your body. Where are your feet? Are
you holding your head in exactly the right way? Is your body
properly aligned?

Initially, this can seem quite difficult and using visualization
techniques can be enormously helpful. By understanding
how your body should be feeling it becomes easier to
assume the correct position. Eventually, these images will
arise naturally through association, without too much effort.

Visualization is one of the best methods to bridge the gap between mind and body. By creating mental pictures that correspond to what you are trying to do physically you will, in time, develop a level of body awareness that is unique to Pilates-based exercises.

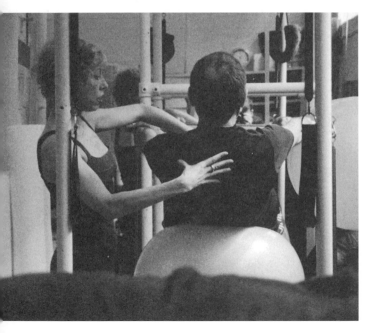

Basic visualization techniques

Anyone can learn to visualize. It helps if you can begin by feeling relaxed. A still mind is more conducive to conjuring up images.

- Spend a few minutes gathering your thoughts. Try to forget about external influences such as work, what you should be doing, and any worries you might have. Remember, this is your time.
- Do some gentle stretches and focus on your breathing. Slow, deep breathing has an instantly calming effect because it helps to promote soothing alpha brain waves. Once you are feeling sufficiently relaxed you can start your exercises.
- As you exercise, focus on each part of your body. How does it feel? With each exercise try to perceive a specific picture. If you are trying to envision yourself on a sandy beach, focus clearly on how this feels. Do your feet feel relaxed, warm, and comfortable? Are your arms hanging loosely by your sides, like a puppet? Where is your head? Think of images that will help you to get into exactly the right position.
- Invite each image to emerge with as much intensity as possible, so that you can almost feel it. Once you have created a familiar picture, eventually all you will have to do is to focus on it and your body will automatically respond.

The aim of Body Maintenance exercises is to bring about permanent changes. You can hasten this process by using visualization techniques when you are not exercising. These will automatically help you to walk, stand, and sit in the correct way.

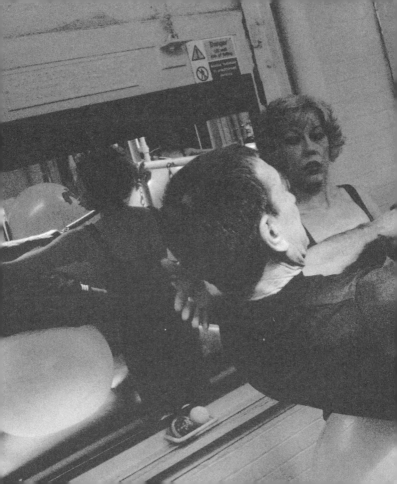

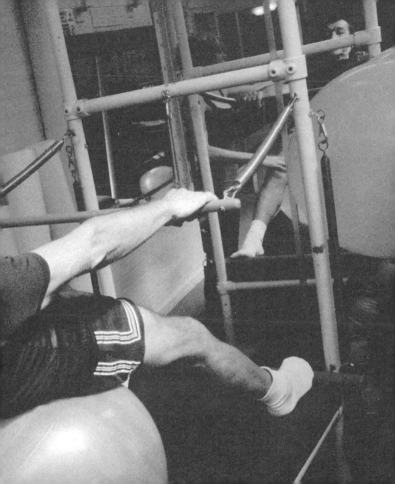

Pilates-based Body Maintenance is a very precise system of exercise. It is different from other regimes in that it requires a bit of groundwork before you start. In order to understand fully what you are doing it is important that you first become acquainted with the basic principles.

essentials

**Before you begin any of the exercises in this book
you must understand and remember the following six
essential guidelines.**

1 Breathing

In dance, a lot of emphasis is placed on the relationship
between breath and movement. However, the importance of
breath is a topic rarely addressed in the gym. Body
Maintenance differs from conventional forms of exercise in
that it concentrates on the correct use of breathing for
each and every exercise.

Breath nourishes the body and the brain. People tend to
breathe shallowly into their upper bodies when they inhale,
into the upper chest and not right down into their lower
lobes. If you are breathing deeply, you're working from the
inside out. You are energizing and replenishing large areas
of your body. Again, it is as much a spiritual as a physical
idea.

For most of the exercises in this book, you will breathe out
on the point of effort. During the exercises think about
oxygen as a rejuvenating life force. Always exhale on the
point of effort. If you have a tight area, try and breathe into
that – breath is another form of liberation, working from the
inside out.

Most people are stronger on one side than on the other, looser on one side and tighter on the other. You are using exercise and breath to create equilibrium in the body.

2 Control

All the exercises in *The Big Little Book of Pilates* are controlled. In this particular instance the word "controlled" means that the correct body parts are being used. Many people, for example, thinking that they are using their abdominals during an exercise, are, in fact using their bones or hip flexors. Thus, the muscles that should be targeted are not being worked in an efficient way.

Control and precision go together. All these exercises are done slowly, in a meditative fashion. You focus the mind on what you're doing, and don't allow it to wander. You use breath, coordination, control, and precision to do a limited number of repetitions well.

You minimize the stress and involvement of other parts of the body. It's preferable to do even five repetitions in a slow and regulated way, than to go through hundreds of motions, during which time nothing effective has happened. In the pelvic tilts, you should be able to feel, literally, one vertebra at a time. The fact that you do 10 repetitions well is better than doing many repetitions badly.

The same principle applies when you are using free-standing weights. In this case, you should be thinking about using internal resistance rather than using your shoulders or snapping your elbows as you use the weights. Focus on the muscles you're using, while making sure that the rest of the body is relaxed and aligned. People often make what is a simple exercise into something quite tortuous, thus creating distortion, tension, and the inability to minimize the movements of other parts of their bodies.

3 Centering

In many Eastern religions, the center of the body is not the heart, but the pelvis. The main principle of the Body Maintenance technique is to recognize that there is one strong, core area that controls the rest of the body. This is located in that part of your body that forms a continuous band at the back and front, between the bottom of your ribcage and across the line of your hipbones. This is called the center. This is the area in which the muscles in your stomach and back are – at the center of your body. These muscles support the internal organs and keep you upright. If you have a strong center you have a strong back, which means you can walk, stand, and run without discomfort or pain. Your arms and legs are extensions of this part of your body. If you have a bad back this is an indication that the center is not strong enough. Originally, human beings were not designed to stand upright. The only reason we stand at all is due to

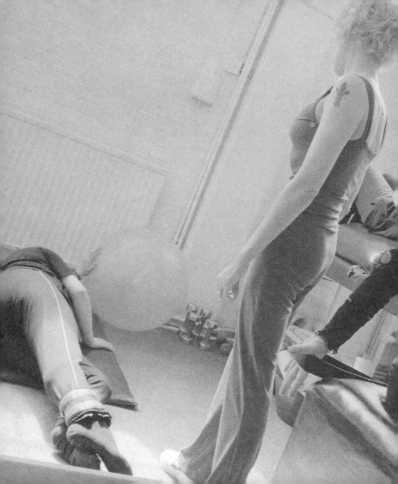

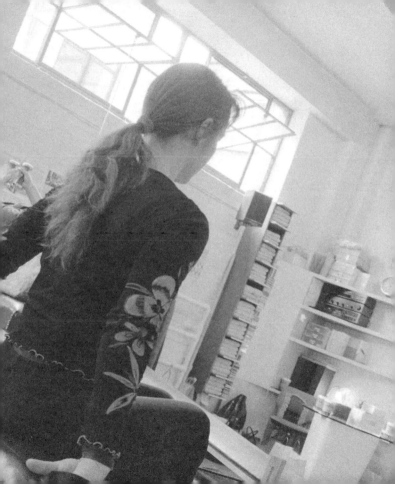

these specific muscles. We are constantly fighting gravity, which pulls us forward. This explains why so many people have all sorts of problems with those muscles affiliated with the shoulders and neck. We are basically defying nature, gravity, and our initial body type.

4 Flow

Each movement in Body Maintenance is designed to be performed in a smooth, flowing, undulating way. There is no room within this regime for any sharp, jarring movements or quick, jerky actions – these are the total antithesis of everything you are trying to achieve. If a movement ever feels like this, you can be sure that you are doing it wrong. Every motion originates from a strong center and flows in a slow, gentle, controlled fashion, thus warming the muscles and causing them to lengthen and open up the spaces between each vertebra in the spine so that the body expands to create a longer, leaner shape.

5 Precision

In order to be effective, all Pilates-based exercises have to be performed with exact precision. This attention to detail is important as it ensures that each movement is working the body in the correct manner. Before you start an exercise sequence, read the instructions carefully. Pay full attention to proper alignment and check what the "watchpoints" have to say. This will ensure that you do not expend excess energy doing an exercise incorrectly.

6 Coordination

Children run naturally, but for most adults basic coordination is a major problem. Many people, when starting Body Maintenance complain to me, "I can't coordinate my breath and the movement. It's too much. I've got to concentrate too hard. I can't do it." Most of us have lost the ability to coordinate the mind and body into a working machine. We no longer have the sense of our feet being in contact with the earth. We've lost the feeling of the way the breath moves naturally through the body. The aim is to retrain the neuromuscular connection between the brain and the body.

This is best illustrated when I try and teach foot exercises to people. I sometimes joke that the feet are very far from the brain and they won't obey, as they haven't been asked to do anything for a long time. Observe people who have lost the use of their hands. They can do the same things with their feet that others can do with their hands. We all have that capability, but we don't employ it. If you don't avail yourself of something it atrophies. Therefore, if you don't use coordination in the physical sense you lose the ability.

Some of the exercises in this book appear quite complicated; that's because they're based upon the introduction of a more complicated concept than mere physical movement. They are trying to reintroduce the mind to the mind/body equation. If I ask my opposite arm and leg to do something at the same time, coordinating from the breath and a strong center, I should be able to achieve it. If I slip in the street, I am more likely to regain my balance than not. If someone throws a bunch of keys at me, I will probably be able to catch it. Because I have the neuromuscular connection between the mind and body parts, I can be spontaneous, and this is where the proprioceptive concept – the linking of mind and body – comes into play.

In *The Big Little Book of Pilates,* we try to re-create your body as a coordinated whole, rather than thinking "I am exercising an arm or leg or the stomach." Coordination is paramount to the way the exercises flow. You might see a Body Maintenance exercise that is similar to those used in aerobic classes or at a gym, but the difference between a Body Maintenance exercise and an aerobic one is that, in Body Maintenance, the movement is concentrated exercise and requires minimal effort from other parts of the body.

KEY TERMS

In Pilates and Body Maintenance there are certain key
terms that are referred to over and over again. It helps if
you understand these before you begin. Also take note of
the special guidance on the feet and neck.

Relaxing

Pilates frequently refers to keeping an area relaxed. This
isn't necessarily what you might think. Most people
associate relaxation with a feeling of "letting go," of
allowing muscles to slump. In this case, to relax means to
release tension in an area while still managing to maintain
tone and control. This should feel comfortable and natural.

Neutral spine

Some of the positions you will be assuming require your spine
to remain in neutral. This means that you maintain the natural
curve in your back. Thus, when you are lying down, do not press
your back so hard into the floor that you lose your natural curve.
Neither must you allow your back to arch so that your lower
back comes off the floor. Just lie there, breathe in and out
naturally, and allow your back to relax into the floor without
pressing it in. This will permit your back to relax into its natural,
neutral position – which is slightly different for everybody.

One vertebra at a time

This refers to one of the main principles that you should
keep in mind whenever you are doing an exercise that

involves rolling your body up from and down to the mat. The idea is that you always roll up gradually so that you are lifting only one vertebra off the mat at a time. The same rule applies when you roll back down again. This takes some practice and initially you will need to concentrate very carefully to ensure that you are doing it correctly.

The center

With Body Maintenance, every exercise originates from the center. The stomach muscles are the core to everything and support the spine. It is important that you always remember to keep this area correctly aligned. This is particularly important when you exercise the lower abdominals as it is very easy to do the opposite of what you actually want. It is natural when you breathe in for the stomach to pull into the spine and when you breathe out for it to bulge. This is not what you want. You will have to try and reverse what the body wants to do unconsciously. As you breathe in you should relax the stomach; as you breathe out you should pull the navel to the spine, engaging the lower abdominal muscles. Your body will naturally want to do the opposite, but it's important to engage the stomach muscles when you exhale.

Straight arms and legs

This is a very common term in Body Maintenance. Your arms and legs should be relaxed and not locked. This is an important point to remember, particularly for the stretches. If an exercise requires that you stretch your arm or leg out straight, you should take care not to overextend, which causes the joints to lock.

The feet

The main thing to remember when exercising is that most of the time you want your feet to be relaxed. If you are in doubt – relax your feet. Most people tense their feet too much and as a result constantly complain about getting cramp in their feet when they are exercising. (If you do get cramp use a foot roller to ease away the tension.) A relaxed foot should feel comfortable, so that there is no sensation of tightness. Whenever you are required to flex your feet, do so by gently stretching out your heel then pulling the top of your foot as far as you can without straining. Do not tense your foot so that it feels strained.

The neck

This is a sensitive part of the body, so you do not want to put it under unnecessary strain while you are exercising. It is very important that you always follow the neck instructions very carefully. Body Maintenance often refers to keeping your neck long, which means adjusting your head into a position that lengthens your neck. When you are doing an exercise lying on your back, the way you bring your head into alignment with the rest of your body is by moving the top of your skull and the base of your neck. Do not attempt to flatten your neck against the floor.

BODY BASICS

The main function of the skeletal system is to provide your body with support, protection, and movement. Bones act as levers and when muscles pull on the bones, this causes parts of the body to move. Muscles are attached to the bones by tendons composed of tough, fibrous, non-elastic connective tissue. The bones you should be most concerned about in Body Maintenance are the main 25 bones that comprise the spinal column, consisting of:

- seven cervical vertebrae in the neck.
- twelve thoracic vertebrae articulating with the ribs in the thorax.
- five lumbar vertebrae in the lower back.
- four bones fused together into the coccyx at the base of the spine.

Movements

All movements involving the bones occur at the joints, thus enabling a variety of different movements. The more common ones that you are likely to come across in Body Maintenance include:

- **flexion** – which bends a limb or the spine, e.g. when bending the head forward onto the chest.
- **extension** – which straightens a limb or the spine.
- **hyperextension** – which means bending back further than the vertical position, e.g. moving the head backwards to look up at the ceiling.

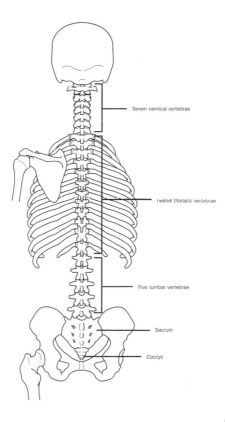

Seven cervical vertebrae

Twelve thoracic vertebrae

Five lumbar vertebrae

Sacrum

Coccyx

- **abduction** – when you make a move away from the center of the body, e.g. raising your arms horizontally sideways.
- **adduction** – when you move towards the center of the body, e.g. you lower your arms to the sides.
- **inversion** – when something turns inwards, e.g. you turn the sole of your foot inwards.
- **rotation** – when the bone turns on its axis either away from or towards the center of the body.

The muscles

Muscles create a movement by exerting a pull on the tendons, which move the bones at the joints. They are also responsible for maintaining posture. Many muscles are attached by the tendons to two articulating bones. Most movements, therefore, involve the use of several muscle groups. Muscles may also work in "antagonistic" pairs – one muscle contracts to move the bone in one direction; the other muscle contracts to move it back, e.g. the calf and shin muscles which raise and lower the foot. Each muscle has the ability to contract or shorten. It can be stretched when it is relaxed. Muscles also control internal functions such as pumping blood round the body and the propulsion of food through the digestive system. There are literally hundreds of muscles in the body (there are 620 muscles that can be consciously controlled alone), all of which are involved in a wide range of functions.

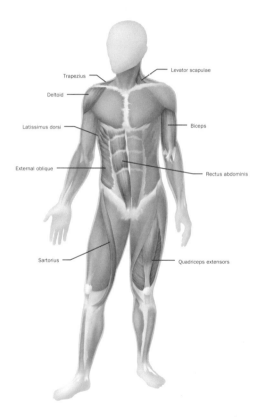

Trapezius

Levator scapulae

Deltoid

Latissimus dorsi

Biceps

External oblique

Rectus abdominis

Sartorius

Quadriceps extensors

The most important muscles you should be aware of for the purposes of Body Maintenance are:

- **trapezius** – in the back of the neck running down to the shoulders.

Action – extends the head.

- **levator scapulae** – at the back and sides of the neck, running into the shoulder.

Action – lifts the shoulder blade and shoulder.

- **deltoid** – on top of the shoulders and upper arms.

Action – moves the arm backwards and forwards.

- **biceps** – at the front of the arms.

Action – moves the arm.

- **triceps** – at the back of the arm.

Action – moves the arm.

- **gluteus maximus** – forms the buttocks.

Action – raises the body, used in running and jumping.

- **gluteus minimus** – in the buttocks.

Action – rotates thigh laterally, maintains balance, used in walking and running.

- **sartorius** – crosses front of thigh from lateral to medial side.

Action – flexes hip and knee, e.g. when sitting cross-legged.

- **semitendinosus (hamstrings)** – down posterior medial side of thigh.

Action – extends thigh, flexes leg at knee.

- **quadriceps extensor** – on the front of the thigh.

Action – opposite movement to hamstrings.

- **external oblique** – extends laterally down the side of the abdomen.

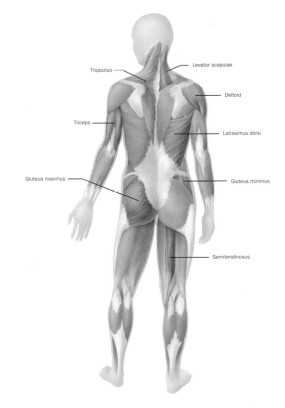

Levator scapulae

Trapezius

Deltoid

Triceps

Latissimus dorsi

Gluteus maximus

Gluteus minimus

Semitendinosus

Action – compresses abdomen, twists trunk.

- **internal oblique** – extends laterally down the side of the front of the abdomen.

Action – compresses abdomen, twists trunk, works with the external oblique.

- **rectus abdominis** – runs down the entire length of the front of the abdomen (divided into four sections).

Action – an important muscle for maintaining posture, draws front of pelvis upwards.

- **transverse abdominis** – runs laterally across front of abdomen.

Action – compresses abdomen.

- **erector spinae** – found medially on the posterior surface of neck, thorax, and abdomen.

Action – extends the spine, holds body upright.

- **latissimus dorsi** – runs down back of lower thorax and lumbar region.

Action – draws shoulders downwards and backwards, adducts and rotates arm, helps pull body up.

BODY AWARENESS

Before you begin any of the Body Maintenance programs, try this simple preliminary body awareness exercise.

Standing or sitting, close your eyes. Take a few deep breaths and, starting with your head, slowly direct your focus down through your entire body. Imagine that you are steering the flow of energy throughout your body. As you do this try to visualize all the different parts of your body along the way. Think of your eyes, ears, mouth, down the shoulders, arms, and hands. Visualize your chest, back, abdomen, hips, pelvic area, upper legs, knees, lower legs, ankles, and feet. As you visit each area try to build up a mental picture of how it looks and feels. Spend a few seconds tuning into each part. Move your head gently, shrug your shoulders. Gently move your stomach, tailbone, and hips. As you do this, concentrate on the sensation. Which areas feel most comfortable and relaxed? Are certain areas tight and constricted? Do this for a few minutes each day. This will help you to become more aware of your body when you are ready to begin the exercises.

The Pilates-based Body Maintenance exercises require total concentration and focus. This makes it particularly important to find a time and place to do them where you know you will not be disturbed.

preparation

In order to be able to concentrate on the exercises it is vital to shut out any other distractions, which may mean switching off the telephone or making sure the children will not disturb you. You will also need to create a specific space for yourself where you can exercise. Most of us do not have the facilities to have our own private gyms! You may, however, find an area in your house that becomes your own retreat. It helps if you get into the right frame of mind. Do this by thinking – this is my time, I am creating a space within my house, within my environment, to work on my body for myself, without distractions.

When to exercise

All the exercises can be done at any time of the day, so choose a time that suits you. If you find it difficult to get going in the mornings, a breakfast session may be just what you need. Alternatively, you might find that you prefer to do them in the early evening, to help you unwind and loosen tight muscles after a busy day. The specific programs on pages 175–217 can also be helpful as they can be slotted into those times of the day when you are under pressure – times when we often most benefit from exercise.

Clothes

Ideally, you should wear clothing in which you can exercise comfortably, such as leggings, shorts, and a T-shirt, or leotard top. Don't wear anything that will restrict your movements. Opt for natural fibers like cotton, which are cooler. You can exercise wearing socks or in bare feet. If you are concerned about slipping, put on a pair of trainers. Take off any jewelry that might get in the way.

Equipment

Having picked a suitable spot in which to exercise, try to create adequate room. This may mean moving the furniture and clearing away any clutter. Before you start, check the floor for any sharp objects or stray pins. Most of the exercises in the core program require little or no equipment. It is essential however to work on a padded surface or a mat. This will protect your spine and prevent any bruising against a hard floor. It is probably worth investing in a proper sports mat. Alternatively, you can work on a folded, synthetic blanket. This should be about five or six feet long and a foot wide. Some of the exercises in the core program involve using props such as a chair, sofa, tennis ball, or towel. If an exercise indicates that you need a couple of light handweights and you don't have any, you can substitute cans of beans. Part Three, Pilates with a Ball, obviously requires a Physio Ball – for advice on these see page 267. If possible, try exercising in front of a full-length mirror. This will enable you to check what you are doing.

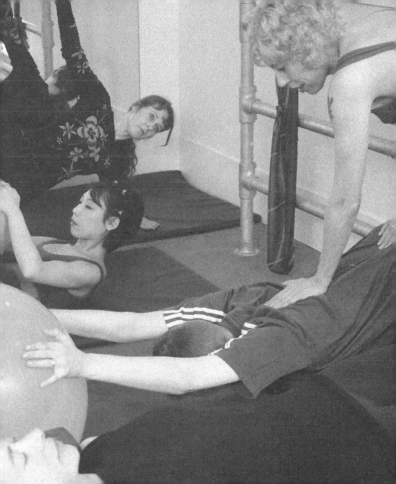

WHICH EXERCISES?

There are two main programs in the book – the core program, which does not rely on any specialist equipment, and the pilates with a ball program, which requires the use of a Physio Ball. Both programs are suitable for all age groups and abilities. However, in many instances using the Physio Ball makes it easier to achieve the correct posture. You can of course mix core program exercises with those using the ball – most of my clients do 25–30 percent of their 90-minute program with the ball. If you do mix the two methods simply stick to the guidelines on sequence set out below. (For more information on the benefits of working with the Physio Balls see the introduction to the program on page 263.)

If you have a specific medical condition such as repetitive strain injury (carpal tunnel syndrome), scoliosis, sciatica, or a bad back, only do those exercises that are recommended for that particular condition *(see Chapter 6)*. If you are pregnant, see Chapter 8.

Sequence of exercises

Begin with the posture and balance exercises or, in the case of the ball exercises, the seated ball exercises. Then move on to the pelvic tilts and the abdominal exercises. It is important to do it in this order, because this way you will be working from a strong center. Even when working your arms and legs, everything is controlled from the center.

Thus, if you are standing and doing a calf stretch, you should be thinking about the location of your stomach, spine, and shoulders. As well as doing some basic abdominal work each session, you should follow strengthening exercises with the relevant stretches. You can then do upper and lower body work on alternate days.

The sequence:
Warm up with the posture and balance exercises or the seated ball exercises.

1 Do all the pelvic tilt and abdominal exercises at the beginning.
2 Proceed to the back exercises.
3 Do leg exercises and stretches.
4 Finish with upper body exercises and stretches.

Read all the instructions carefully. Remember the breathing instructions.

Continue to add exercises each day as you feel more comfortable. Use your own judgement. If you are unsure do the pelvic tilts and abdominal exercises, then add to them. If you feel any discomfort in your back during any particular exercise, you still have insufficient core strength to do it.

The following safety rules will help:

- Always do stretches after the relevant strengthening exercises.
- Do not attempt to do too much too soon. Increase the number of repetitions gradually.
- Always stop if you feel nauseous, fatigued, or extremely breathless.
- If you have any chest pains (especially when accompanied by pain in the arm, neck, shoulders, and jaw) – stop exercising immediately and seek medical help.
- If exercise leaves you unnaturally tired, check with your physician.
- The neck is a sensitive area of the body. If you cannot remember whether you have worked this area or not, it is better not to do any further repetitions.
- Always make sure that there is something you can hold on to for support when doing the balancing exercises.
- If you experience back pain – stop.
- If your muscles start shaking – stop.
- Drink plenty of fluids afterwards, especially when it is hot.

Before you embark on any new program, it's a good idea to consult your physician. A pre-exercise check-up is strongly advised if you are over 40 or have not been exercising regularly. Always seek the advice of a specialist if you have a medical condition, are pregnant, or have any chronic joint problems.

PART TWO

practical pilates

The exercises in this section will help you to tone and strengthen specific muscles in your arms, back, stomach, chest, and legs. In time, as your body adapts, you will also start to look taller, slimmer, and more youthful.

4

the core exercise program

Before you attempt any of the exercises in the rest of
the core program, start with the following essential
posture and balance exercises. It is best to do these
in bare feet. If you've got a mirror – even better. That
way, if you stand sideways, you'll be able to keep an
eye on what you're doing and make sure that it's
correct.

HOW TO LOOK INSTANTLY TALLER AND SLIMMER

Not sure if you're standing correctly? Then practice the
position on the following page for a few minutes daily. After
a while it will feel so natural that you no longer have to
think about it.

posture and balance exercises

Stand with your feet hip-width apart. Imagine that you're standing on sand. Your feet are relaxed. Think of your weight being over the middle of each foot, with your toes gently lengthening into the sand. Close your eyes and make a mental note of the following.

- Don't sink back into your heels or lean forward. Keep your weight evenly distributed over your feet.
- Let your arms fall naturally in front of your body.
- Let your hands hang from the shoulders, totally loose and relaxed.
- Don't lock your knees. They should feel relaxed and not rigid.
- Keep your inside thighs and bottom relaxed.
- Imagine that your head is like one of those nodding dogs in the back of a car. It's not going backwards and forwards but resting directly upon your shoulders and rocking gently until it settles into a comfortable, neutral position.
- Think of the bones directly behind your ears. Try to imagine them "reaching" towards the ceiling.
- Pull your stomach in, without tipping the pelvis forward. Think of a piece of string from your pubic bone to your navel. It is shortening as you pull up and in. Feel your tailbone drop – as if it is weighted to the floor. This will seem much easier after you've done more of the stretches to release the pelvic girdle.
- Keep the front of your thighs relaxed.

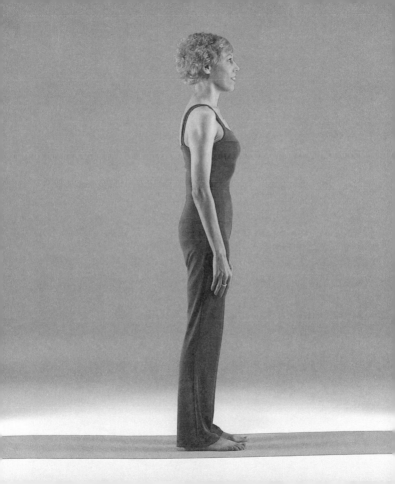

Now your whole body is perfectly aligned – you should feel as if you are floating an inch off the ground.

EXERCISES FOR BETTER BALANCE

If you're worried about slipping, tripping, or not being able to catch objects thrown towards you, your sense of balance is probably poor. What seems to occur, as you get older or as a result of any injury, is that you lose your awareness of balance and your reflexes are no longer as sharp. This can cause great feelings of insecurity. Perhaps you begin to worry more about safety. We all know that the simplest of falls might have serious consequences. This is reflected in the body, which becomes stiff and constricted as a result. The easiest way to change this is to practice the following exercises every day. In time, you will start to feel lighter and more confident in the way you move.

For each of these exercises all the same rules as the "perfect posture" exercise apply (see the checklist on page 68).

- With bare feet, stand on both legs, and imagine you are on a beach with soft sand between your toes. Let one foot float off the ground.
- Count for 10 seconds and change legs. Repeat four times, twice on each leg.
- Now do the same – with your eyes closed. Make sure you have something to hold on to, lest you fall over.

Standing on one leg on a towel

Do exactly the same as in the exercise above, standing on a flat towel. This gives you a slightly more unstable surface and makes the exercise more difficult. Even if you don't regularly exercise, try to do these every day – especially if you are over 45.

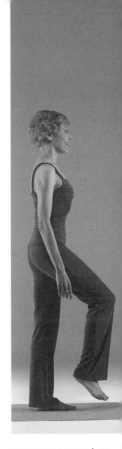

Start in the "perfect posture" position and, with feet approximately an inch apart, start to walk backwards. Slowly drag your foot back, so that it never entirely leaves the floor. The easiest way to master this is to imagine that you are trying to remove some chewing gum from under your feet.

Look in the mirror – but do not look down at your feet. This exercise is even more effective if you imagine you are walking on sand.

BREATHING

Correct breathing is a very important facet of Pilates. By remembering to breathe properly, you'll find it becomes much easier to exercise. The problem is that most people don't breathe deeply enough. Breathing slowly and deeply is very energizing. It ensures there is sufficient oxygen circulating throughout the body.

It may sound obvious, but when you exercise do not hold your breath. It's better to breathe incorrectly than not at all. Practice the following exercise before you start any of the stomach work.

- Lie on your back in a relaxed position, resting your head on a folded towel, with your knees bent.
- Place one hand on your stomach and, very gently, breathe in through your nose. Feel your lungs filling with oxygen and slowly expand and relax your stomach. Breathe out.
- With one finger on your pubic bone and one on your navel, try to shorten that gap as you breathe out, and flatten your stomach to your spine without tilting your pelvis.
- Breathe in again and feel that gap slightly expand.
- Breathe out. Imagine there is a piece of string or an elastic band that links your pubic bone to your navel. Very gently feel it pulling up and in. This will get all three sets of stomach muscles working, including your oblique muscles, which will tighten your waist.

Make sure you breathe slowly and deeply. One of the main rules of Pilates is to breathe out on the point of effort. If in doubt, particularly on the stretches – breathe naturally.

When you breathe in your stomach gently expands. However, it shouldn't swell in an exaggerated way. Try and think of your ribcage expanding gently to the sides so that you're not just breathing into your throat and upper chest.

When you begin the exercise program and you start to breathe properly you might feel a bit dizzy. As you are learning to breathe more deeply, you are taking in more oxygen, which can make you feel light-headed.

Women are often obsessed with having flat stomachs like men, regardless of the obvious physical differences. These exercises, combined with careful and healthy eating, will tone and tighten the stomach area. They will not make you lose weight, but they will give you a flatter, leaner stomach.

As people age, their metabolism changes and they must exercise more to burn up the same amount of calories. By exercise, I mean walking instead of taking the car, or climbing the stairs instead of taking the elevator. If you're short-waisted and eat large meals, you are going to have a stomach that protrudes. It is better for your blood sugar levels to eat small amounts of complex carbohydrates throughout the day. Also allow yourself some flexibility, and don't obsessively deny yourself certain foods.

In Pilates when you do your abdominal work, as you breathe in the stomach gently expands. As you breathe out the stomach pulls in, navel to spine. Feel the connection from the pubic bone up to the navel. The body will automatically want to do the opposite as you breathe out on the point of effort. You inhale through the nose and exhale through the mouth. As you breathe out think about pulling the navel to the spine without tipping the pelvis. If you have trouble with the pelvis and you have tight hip flexors and glutes, go to the section of the leg stretches where you stretch your bottom with the foot on the thigh *(see page 131),* and do one or two of those stretches first to relax your pelvis.

A strong stomach exists to support your internal organs and back. The taller you stand, the more balanced your stance, the flatter your stomach will appear. When you are posturally aligned and maintaining an erect back while walking, you are exercising your body perfectly well. If you sit slouched all the time and if you walk with a slump, your stomach will stick out. These abdominal and back exercises are good for conditioning, toning, and strengthening. They're also good for anyone with a bad back, sciatica, or scoliosis. If you have any of these problems you need to do abdominal and back work, but try the remedial exercises in Chapter 6 before moving on to the exercises in this section.

It's better to do these exercises either lying on a towel or on an exercise mat. As you're lying on your back, you may want to place a folded towel under your head. This will help lengthen your neck. If you're not sure about this, try it with and without to see which is more comfortable.

Repeat each exercise 10 times. Do the stretches in sets of four. Stomach muscles have an unusually short memory. Daily reminders will keep them taut and toned.

The pelvic tilt is a preparation exercise that warms up the back. It's a good starting point, whatever part of the program you plan to do.

Lie on your back, with your knees bent and parallel, about hip-width apart. Arms should be resting at your sides, with palms facing the floor. This helps to lengthen your neck. Breathe in, then breathe out and gently relax your back into the floor. When you do this, do not press your back too strongly to the ground so that you lose your natural curve. Do not allow your back to arch to the point that it lifts off the floor. This is called the neutral spine position and it is slightly different for everybody *(see page 47)*. There is no point in trying to force your back down. Try very hard not to tense your buttock muscles during this exercise.

As you breathe out, gently tilt your pelvis forward and roll your lower back off the floor – one vertebra at a time, as you "peel" your back off the mat *(see page 47)*. Breathe in, keeping your neck long, and very slowly roll all the way down, breathing out. Keep your feet relaxed on the floor and imagine that your toes are "lengthening" away.

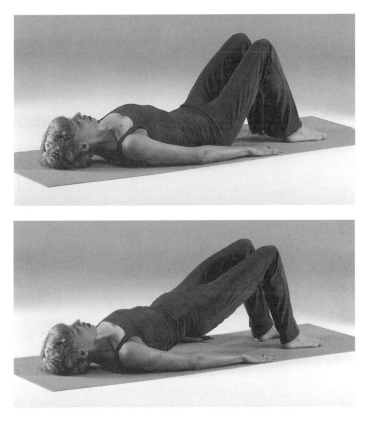

This is a preparation for the abdominal exercises. It will wake up your stomach muscles and prepare you for the more difficult exercises.

Lie as before – with a relaxed back and long neck, without tucking the pelvis under. Take either a small cushion or folded towel and place it between your thighs. Very gently breathe in through your nose. As you breathe out, feel your stomach muscles pulling down to the floor. Think of them pulling up and into your spine. Hold your breath and count to four. Squeeze the towel or cushion with your thighs. You can put your fingers on your stomach if you wish so that you can feel the muscles you are working.

As you breathe in through your nose, feel your stomach gently expand into your fingers. As you breathe out, feel your stomach pull away from your fingers. Feel your lower abdominal muscles working. Think of working on the transverse and the rectus abdominis muscles first, and the obliques second. Repeat 10 times.

Watchpoints

■ Don't let your pelvis lift off the floor. This will "shorten" the neck. Watch that your stomach doesn't "bloat." Instead, make sure that on the point of relaxation – when you breathe in – the stomach gently lifts. As you breathe out you should feel your stomach pull up and in, away from the pubic bone.

■ Most people naturally want to breathe in and pull their stomach muscles in – this is a mistake. As you breathe in, you gently soften the muscles as they flow out into your fingers. As you breathe out the stomach pulls away from the fingers. Think of it as pulling "up and in." This will help you focus on your lower abdominals – strengthening and toning that area.

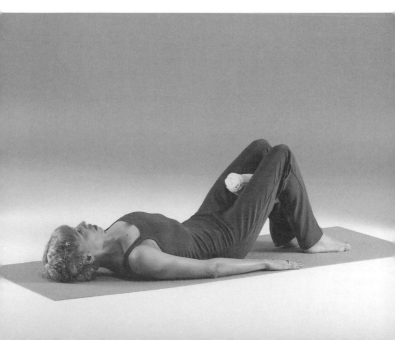

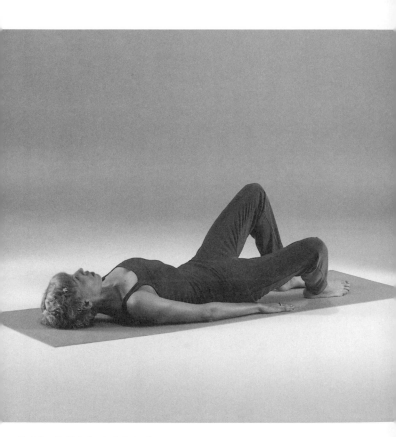

Lie in the same position as in the previous exercise, knees bent. Place your hands on your hipbones. This helps to stabilize your pelvis. Begin with the right leg. Keep your left leg completely still. Very gently breathe in and let your right knee open sideways. As you breathe out feel the resistance. Bring the leg back to the other one – breathing out and pulling your stomach in. Change legs. Now, breathing in, open the left leg to the side. Exhale and slowly close. Repeat 10 times, alternating legs each time.

Watchpoints

■ Think of the muscles between your navel and your pubic bone as a fan. As you inhale and the knee opens to the side the fan opens. As you exhale, the muscles tighten and the fan closes.

■ Don't tilt the pelvis, and make sure that the supporting side is stable.

■ Don't press your back into the mat.

This slightly harder version of the previous exercise is very straightforward. Interlace your hands behind your head. (This will help prevent you from straining the muscles in your neck.) Slide them high up behind your skull. Do not let them slip to the neck. Keep your thumbs on either side of your spine.

Lift your elbows so that you can just see them out of the corner of your eye without moving your head. When you can see your elbows peripherally you know that your arms are in the right place. Very gently exhale and "float" your head and shoulders off the mat. Hold that position and repeat the previous exercise. Repeat the exercise 10 times, five times on each side.

Watchpoint

- As you lift your head, your focus shouldn't change, so you don't shorten your neck. If you shorten your neck you may tip your pelvis. This makes it very hard to work your lower abdominal muscles. You may also place a strain on your lower back and your body will be incorrectly aligned.

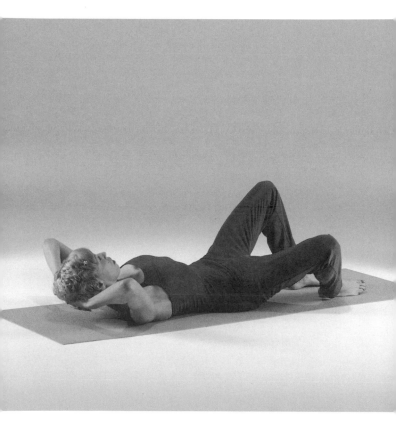

This exercise uses exactly the same position as the previous exercise, although the knee does not fan out. All the same rules apply. Lift your elbows up to where you can see them in your peripheral vision. Keep looking at the ceiling and gently breathe in through your nose. Relax the abdomen, but do not "bloat" it out. As you breathe out, gently lift your head and shoulders off the mat. Only go as high as you can. Do not strain your neck to hold that position. Breathe in as you go back down again.

Watchpoint

- As you breathe out, imagine that a piece of string is pulling you up from your pubic bone and under your rib cage. Pause until all three sets of abdominal muscles go "up and in," and flatten.

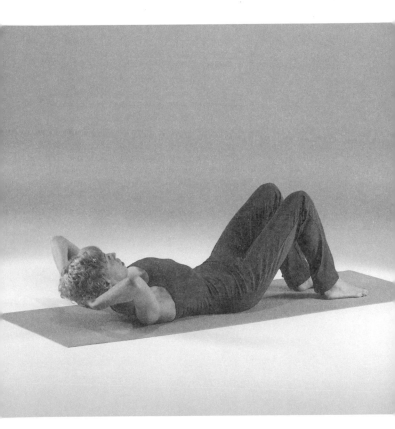

This stomach exercise is a simple single leg stretch. It is the first really coordinated exercise. It is a simple and basic exercise – which is not the same as saying it is easy.

Start in the same position as the previous exercises and interlace your hands behind your head. Lift your head and shoulders gently off the mat. As you breathe out, slide your right leg down, an inch off the floor. Breathe in, putting your head down and bringing your right leg back up. Breathe out, and slide your left leg down, an inch off the floor. Repeat 10 times, alternating legs.

Watchpoints

- Many people make the mistake of exhaling before curling forward. If you do this, you will not get the same benefit. You exhale as you do the exercise.

- Remember to keep looking at that same point on the ceiling. If you pull your chin into your chest you may strain your neck and won't get the results you want.

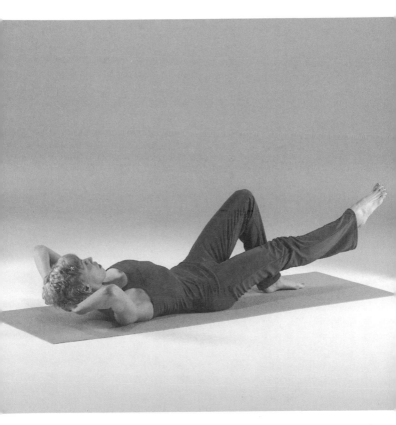

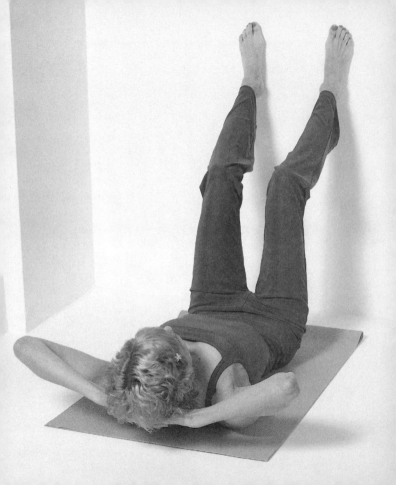

Lie on your back with your legs comfortably against a wall
or with your feet held up by a friend. Be close enough to, or
far enough away from, the wall so that your tailbone is
weighted to the mat. If your bottom is off the ground you're
too close to the wall. Conversely, if you're too far away your
legs won't feel supported.

Take your hands behind your head and lift your elbows to
where you can see them in your peripheral vision. Keep the
neck long.

Very gently breathe in to prepare. As you breathe out, lift
the head and shoulders off the mat, pulling your stomach
towards your spine. Pause, breathe in, and lower. As you
breathe out and lift, the stomach pulls in, the pelvis does
not lift. The neck is long, the head is cradled in the hands.
You are not pulling your chin to your chest. Think of the
breast bone and the head as floating off the mat. Don't
think of a sharp pulling movement.

Do 10 repetitions.

Watchpoint

- Hands are interlaced high up behind the cranium and are not
  placed behind the neck.

This is the most difficult exercise in the program, because it is an exercise with both legs off the ground. If you have any back injuries at all, don't do it until you feel strong enough.

Bend both knees into the chest and allow your tailbone to be relaxed and heavy. Your hands are linked behind your head as before. Look at the ceiling and breathe out. Let your head and shoulders "float" off the ground, depending on how much mobility you have. Inhale.

Exhale and stretch one leg out, pulling your stomach into the spine. Inhale and bring the leg back. Exhale and extend the other leg. Do five stretches on each leg. If you wish you may relax at the end and do another set. Only take the leg as low as the point where your back does not arch away from the floor. The lower the leg, the harder the exercise.

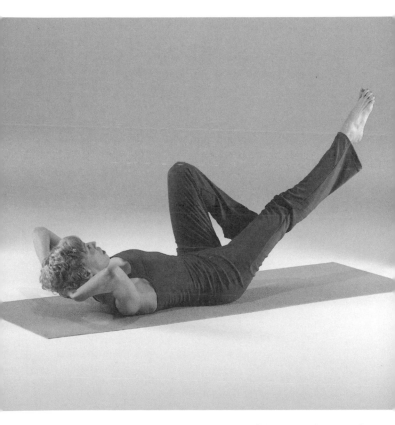

The next three exercises are also for the abdomen but they are done lying on your side. These are called side stretches and side lifts. They are particularly good for the waist obliques. The same rules apply as for all the abdominal exercises. It doesn't matter which side you lie on to start with. Do all the exercises in sets of 10. The rest of the exercises in this section are for the back.

You cannot stand upright if you have a tight, weak back. Any minor adjustments that you make to try to correct the way in which you walk, sit, and stand will only create further problems. Gentle exercise and control are the key. If you envision these exercises as stomach exercises, you can't go wrong. If you think of them as back exercises, the result will be frenetic movement that won't accomplish much except possibly "concertina-ing" your bones.

If time allows, these lower back exercises should be done after the stomach exercises. These exercises work better as a pair. You must strengthen your stomach before you start working on your back, as the abdominal muscles initiate the work needed to develop a strong back. All exercises are directed from the abdominals.

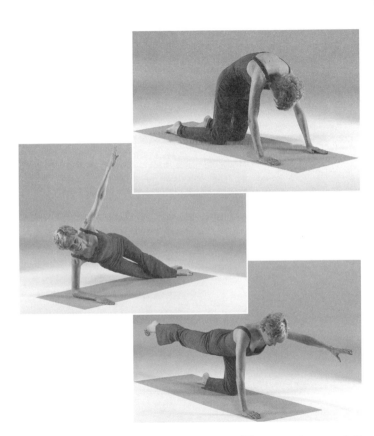

Lie on your side, arm stretched out in line with your body,
palm down. Place your other hand on the floor in front of
you, for balance. If your neck doesn't feel comfortable,
place a folded towel between your ear and your shoulder.
Think of your ear "lengthening" along the arm, so that you're
looking directly ahead of you. The hips are stacked one directly
over the other so that your pelvis is level, not tilted. It's very
common to let the top hip rock forward. Glance down your body
without moving your head. If you can't see your feet, they are
too far behind you. If you feel any strain in your back, the first
thing you should do is move your feet further forward.

Breathe in to prepare. Breathe out and lift your legs about
four inches off the ground. Keep your feet gently flexed. You
want to straighten the back of your legs. Feel the energy
pushing through your heels as you lift. Breathe in as you
lower. Do 10 on each side.

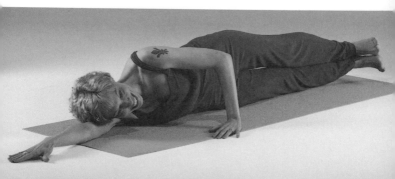

Watchpoints

■ If you are unsure about this position, do it with your back against the wall. You can then feel how far your legs have to come forward to feel your middle back against the wall.

■ Stretch your legs as far as you can without locking your knees. The knees are lengthened away, but slightly relaxed. If you're not sure about locking your knees or stretching your knees it's always better to have them slightly released.

side stretch 2

The next exercise is simply a harder version of the one before – so all the same rules apply. Use a towel if you need to. Relax your top arm and shoulder. With flexed feet breathe out and think of your legs floating off the ground. Hold this position and breathe in. Breathe out and lift the top leg. Bring the leg back, breathe in, and slowly lower both legs to the ground and relax. Do 10 repetitions on each side.

Watchpoints

■ It's really important for this exercise that you never allow one leg to become longer than the other. You don't want an imbalance in your pelvis.

■ Correct breathing is vital. If you feel any strain in your back, try doing the exercise with your legs further forward.

This exercise is more difficult and you need to be reasonably fit to try it. Don't attempt it if you have any back injuries.

Lie on your side, with your elbow directly under your shoulder, your palm flat on the floor. Keep your legs in a straight line with your ankles crossed. It helps if you can place your feet against a hard surface – e.g., a skirting board, or the bottom of a sofa. This will give you a bit of resistance and help you get off the ground. All the same rules on alignment apply as in the side stretch. Keep your shoulder and elbow in line. As you breathe out, lift, pushing down through the supporting arm. The other arm lifts up to a right angle in line with the shoulder. Come back down again and relax. Begin by doing this exercise four times on each side and slowly build up to 10. This will give you a strong, toned, and, hopefully, very trim waist.

Watchpoint

- Don't allow the top arm to swing behind you. This is a common fault and can cause the body to rock backwards.

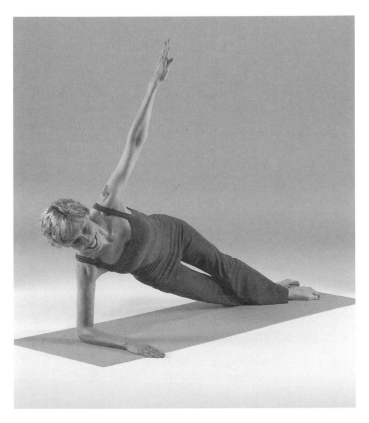

A cat stretch is done on your hands and knees. Make a square of your body. Keep your hands under your shoulders, fingers facing forwards and with your hands shoulder-width apart. Knees should be hip-width apart. If your knees feel a bit uncomfortable, just fold up a towel and put it under them. Place your feet gently on the floor and don't lock your elbows at any point. As you breathe out, drop your chin to your chest and curl your stomach into the spine. Press your upper back to the ceiling, trying not to rock back and forth. As you breathe in, your tailbone lifts towards the ceiling, your chest presses to the floor, and your head gently lifts. Breathe out and reverse the position. After 10 repetitions, relax your bottom onto your heels and just breathe. This is called the "relaxation position." You can do this relaxation at the end of the sequence of back exercises, or at the end of each back exercise.

Watchpoints

- Don't lock your elbows.

- Don't lift your head too high or you may strain your neck.

- As you press your chest down to the floor (in the reverse exercise), if you feel any pinching in your lower back you'll know you've gone too far.

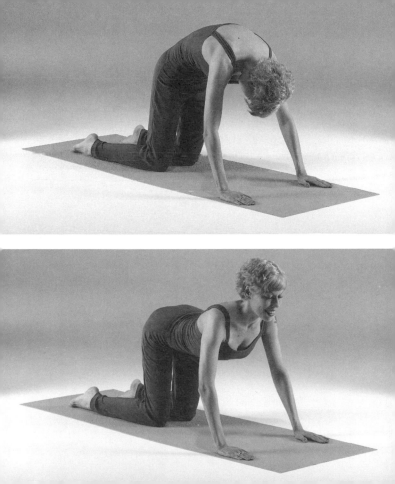

Lie on your stomach with your feet relaxed. Your arms
should be facing forwards and be just wider than your
shoulders, which are relaxed. Keep your neck "long" by
looking down. Keep looking down as you gently press your
hips and elbows into the floor and pull your stomach in.
Gently, lift your head up (keep it independent of the body),
focusing your eyes on the same point. Make sure you keep
your feet on the floor. Breathe in, and gently come down.
Feel your buttocks contract slightly. Do not contract them

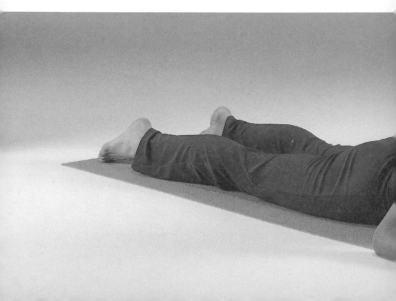

too much – otherwise you're using your buttock muscles and not the stomach. Engaging the abdominals helps to strengthen your back and lift your body.

As you breathe out and lift, imagine that the crown of your head is going forward towards the wall in front of you. Do not lift your head towards the ceiling. Ideally, you want as little pressure on the hands as possible. Relax your fingers and feel your shoulder blades releasing. Relax down again.

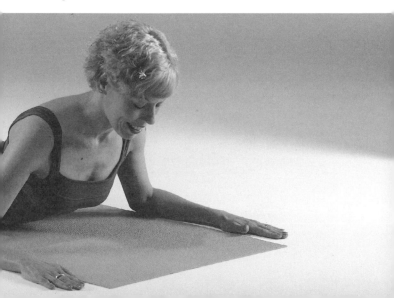

This exercise is exactly the same as the previous one, except that this time, as you breathe out and lift, your hands "float" off the ground.

Watchpoints

- As you breathe out and lift, you should be able to get your fingers between your stomach and the floor.

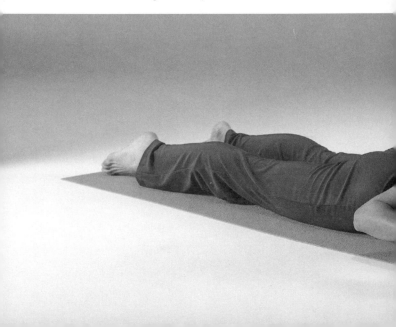

- Whenever you do a back exercise, each time you breathe out, your stomach goes into the spine (just as in the earlier abdominal exercises). If you lift too high and you feel your back shortening, you've gone too far.

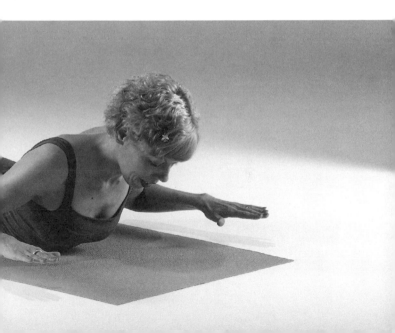

This works your stomach and your back.

Lying on your stomach, imagine yourself in the shape of
a rather small starfish. Your arms are slightly wider than
your shoulders. Look down at the floor. Make sure your
legs are comfortably apart and rotated slightly outwards.
Don't force it though, simply lie there and just let your
legs relax into their natural position. Exhale and let your
left leg and right arm gently float off the ground. Feel
your stomach doing all the work. Breathe in and lower.
Exhale as you change sides. Make sure that as your

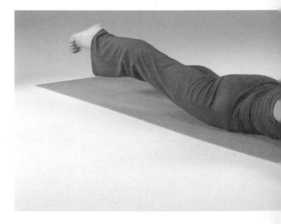

stomach goes in your tailbone drops. As you breathe,
don't grip your bottom. Again, keep your legs straight and
shoulders relaxed. Your arms and legs should be at the
same height. Repeat 10 times, alternating between
sides.

Watchpoint

- Don't shorten your neck, grip your bottom, or lift your arm
  and leg too high. Don't think of "lifting" – you should be
  "lengthening" your arm and leg. The idea here is to do a
  diagonal stretch that strengthens and mobilizes the big back
  muscle between the base of one shoulder blade and the top
  of the opposite buttock.

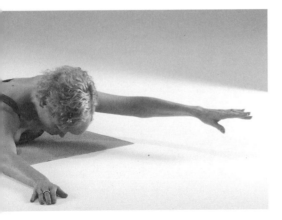

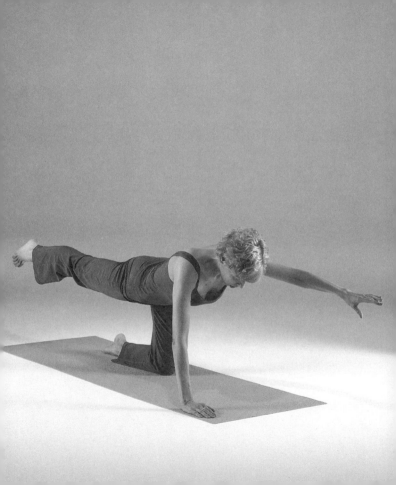

This exercise helps improve balance.

Assume the same position as the cat stretch *(see page 98)*. The spine is neutral and stomach gently in. Imagine someone's hand on your stomach. Breathe out, and let your right arm and left leg gently float away. Don't lift too high. To avoid this, position something like a kitchen roll across the base of your spine. If you lift too high, it will fall off. Keep your pelvis neutral, so that you don't tilt from side to side. Keep looking at the same point on the floor, so that you don't shorten your neck. Relax back into the starting position. Repeat, alternating arms and legs for 10 repetitions.

Watchpoint

- If this exercise feels too difficult at the onset, you can start by lifting one arm, or one leg only.

All the same rules apply as in the alternate arm and leg
stretch *(see page 104)*. Once again, imagine you are a
small starfish, lying on your front, with your arms and legs
comfortably apart. As you breathe out, simultaneously lift
both arms and both legs to the same height. Keep looking
down throughout, and pull your stomach into your spine
until you feel your tailbone drop.

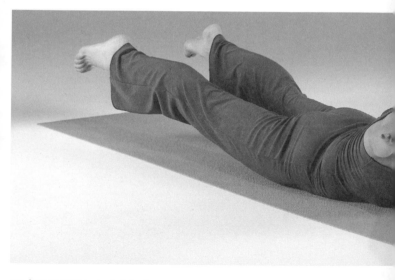

Watchpoints

■ Make sure that as your stomach goes in, your pelvis relaxes back; as you breathe, don't grip your bottom.

■ Again, keep your legs straight. If you bend your knees the exercise won't be effective.

■ Keep shoulders relaxed, stomach in, legs and arms straight. Your arms and legs should be at the same height.

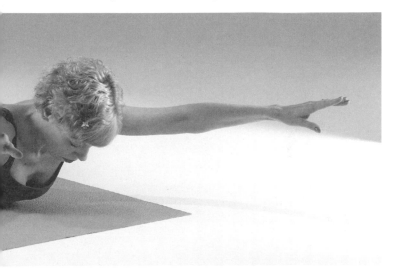

Do this at the end of the back exercise sequence.

Sit back down on your heels with your arms close to your sides. Gently pull your head into your chest and curl yourself into a small "ball" until your forehead touches the ground. Hold for a few seconds.

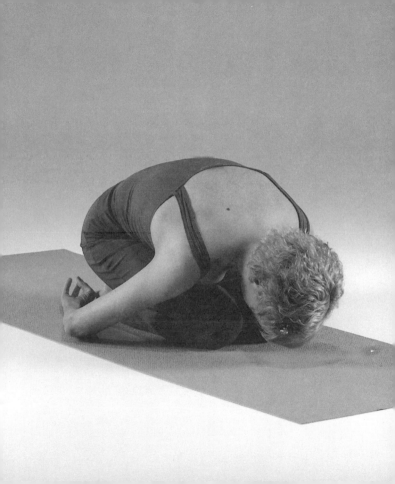

It is possible to create bulk by exercising the legs if you do not do enough stretching. Everyone wants their leg muscles to be long, lean, and lengthened as opposed to tight and bunched. There are certain parts of the legs, particularly the quadriceps muscles above the knees, that get bigger due to excessive use, while the inside thighs and the hamstrings are usually undertoned. Many people tend to have overdeveloped quads, weak inside thighs and tight, but not strong, hamstrings.

The following exercises will help to strengthen, tone, and condition your legs and help to make them more shapely.

Any of the following exercises can be done with ankle weights. However, don't use anything heavier than two pounds/one kilo. You want to tone and lengthen muscles, not build them up.

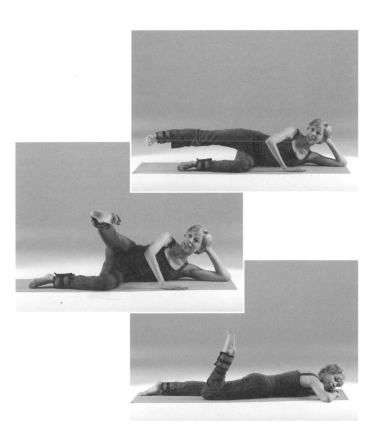

This exercise will help tone flabby inside thighs.

You can do this lying on your side, either with your hand supporting your head, or with your arm completely flat. If you choose to keep your arm flat, it may feel more comfortable to put a towel between your arm and ear. Your top leg should be forward, in front of the body. If this feels awkward, place a pillow under your knee. The other hand is in front of you. The underneath leg (the one that is working) needs to be slightly forward, with your foot gently flexed. Again, don't lock your knee, but pull up the muscles, so that your leg is straight. If your legs are not straight, you'll be working your ankle and your foot much more than your inside thigh.

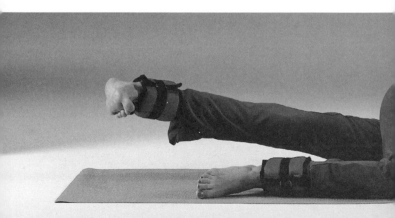

Breathe out, lift your leg, and hold. Then slowly lower it. Don't lift your leg too high. Think of your leg going "away," not up – as you want to lengthen and strengthen your muscles, not have them contracted and tight. As you lift and breathe out, your stomach pulls in, just like in the earlier stomach exercises. The energy is through the heel, working your inside thigh. Do 10 on each side.

Watchpoint

- It's important to remember that, in all the leg exercises, the instigator is your stomach. This means you should feel your abdominal muscles working. The same applies to all the upper body exercises.

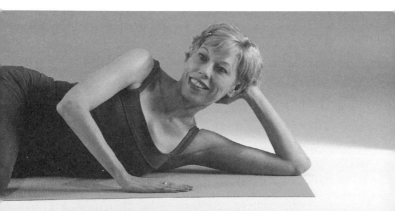

Assume the same position as in the previous exercise. Gently point your foot. Breathe out and lift your leg. Slowly circle the leg in each direction. As you circle the leg, don't think of going up and down. Think of going out and away, so that you're almost touching the floor, as if you're circling around a coin.

Do 10 little circles each way on each leg.

Watchpoint

- The knee is gently pulled up, the leg is reaching away, and you're circling down and away, not up.

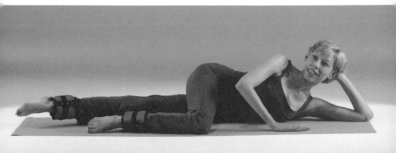

This works the outer thighs and buttocks.

Take up the same position as before, only this time your underneath leg is bent comfortably in front of you. The top leg is straight, flexed, and very slightly forward. If you've got any doubts about your back arching, you can lean against a wall.

The top leg should start the exercise at hip height. Very gently breathe out and lift the leg about six inches. Don't turn your toes towards the ceiling. Keep your foot facing forward, gently flexed. When you breathe out and lift, focus on the outer thigh and the back of the leg.

Do 10 on each side.

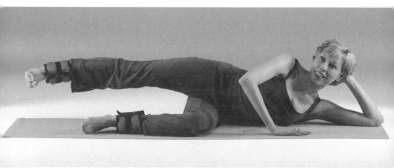

Start this exercise in the same position as the outer thigh lift. Make sure your top heel is in line with your hip. Very gently breathe out and bring your leg forward, so that it's in line with the other knee. Breathe in, and lift. Breathe out, and lower and take the leg back. This is quite a demanding exercise, so start with five on each side, then gradually build up to 10.

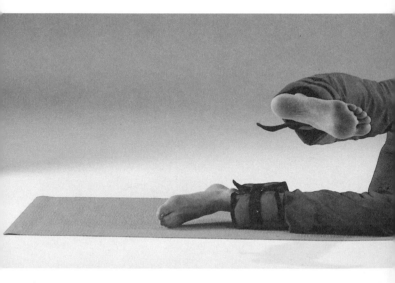

Watchpoints

■ As you breathe out and pull your leg forward, don't swing it. Think of your leg as a "resistance," so that it is the stomach that is bringing your leg forward, up, down, and back, as you tone the back of the thigh. Keep it in line with the other knee. Your hip stays back, your stomach stays in.

■ If you find you get cramp in your hip, this exercise might not be for you.

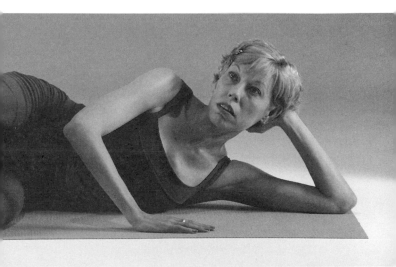

In the same position as the previous exercise, bend both
knees, so that they are comfortably in front of you. Gently
flex your feet. Lift the top leg, as if you're opening a fan.
Then very gently breathe out, and squeeze the top leg to
straight. As you breathe in, make a small bend in the knee.
Breathe out and squeeze to straight. Remember – the

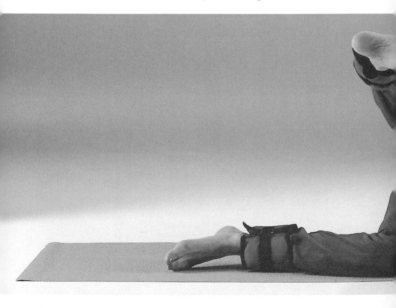

emphasis is not on the bend, but on the squeeze. If you do a big bend, you'll be working your calves, not your bottom. Do 10 on each side.

Watchpoint

■ If you get cramp, this indicates that your muscles are fatigued and it is best to stop.

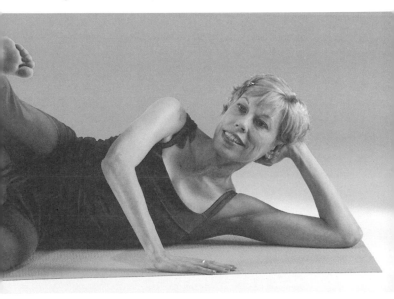

Lying on your stomach, your head should be comfortably
relaxed on your hands. If you prefer, keep your arms at your
sides. Do whichever feels more comfortable. Keep your
shoulders relaxed. Very gently "grip" your bottom. As you do
so, you should feel your stomach going in and your tailbone
drop. Inhaling, bend your right leg and flex your foot. Then
gently exhale and straighten, keeping the buttocks squeezed
at all times. Repeat 10 times then change legs. (The bend
on this exercise is not important, it's just a preparation.)

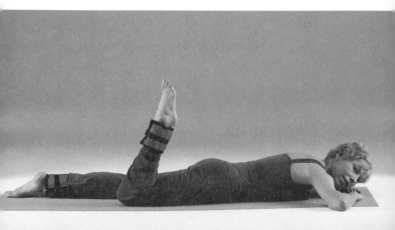

Assume the same position on your stomach as in the
previous exercise. With a straight leg, hip down, stomach
in, keeping foot relaxed, very gently breathe out and lift your
leg up. Then slowly bring it down. This works the buttock
muscles, which are just under the cheek. Do 10 repetitions
on each leg.

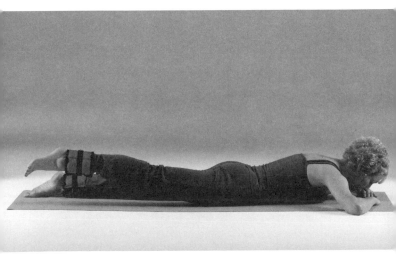

This is exactly the same as the previous exercise, except this time as you breathe out and lift, keep your foot softly flexed. Repeat 10 times on one leg and then the other.

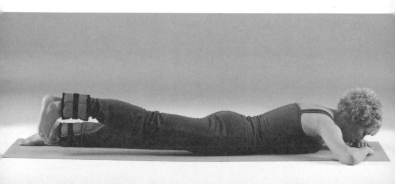

This is the last exercise in this sequence, and all the same rules apply as before. Starting in the same position, this time you bend your leg and flex your foot as you lift. Keep your hip down, and foot, knee, and ankle in line, as you breathe out and slowly squeeze towards the ceiling.

Repeat 10 times on one leg and then the other.

Watchpoints

- At no point in any of the three bottom toner exercises should your hipbones leave the mat.

- If you feel your back arch, place a rolled towel beneath your stomach.

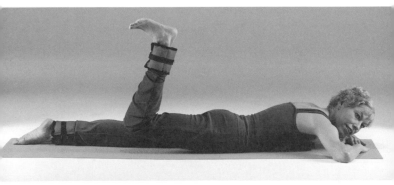

leg stretches

It is vital that you do leg stretches after you've done any leg
strengthening work. They are especially important if you
have any back problems. If you've got a tight back, you may
have tight legs. Sometimes it's difficult to know which
comes first – a bad back and tight hamstrings, or tight
hamstrings resulting in a bad back. Also, if you do have
back problems you are likely to have a pelvic imbalance,
which is often caused by over-tight gluteal muscles, hip
flexors, and quadriceps, so that your pelvis is not in line.
If you can get your body in line, you'll feel much more
comfortable, and you will avoid a lot of problems.

Hold all stretches for 30 seconds.

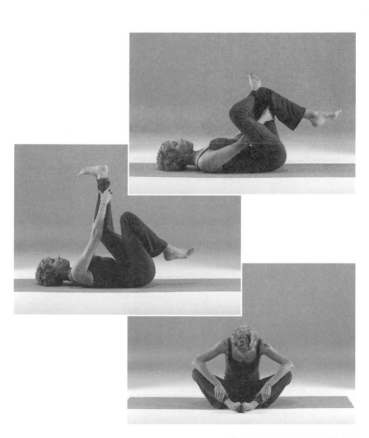

Lying down on your back, cross your knees, hold onto your ankles, and very gently pull your heels into your bottom. Do this for 30 seconds with the right leg on top, then 30 seconds with the left leg on top. Repeat four times in total.

Watchpoints

- Don't let your bottom lift – it should stay "weighted" to the ground.

- Don't hold onto your feet – hold onto your ankles.

- If it feels more comfortable, place a towel under your head.

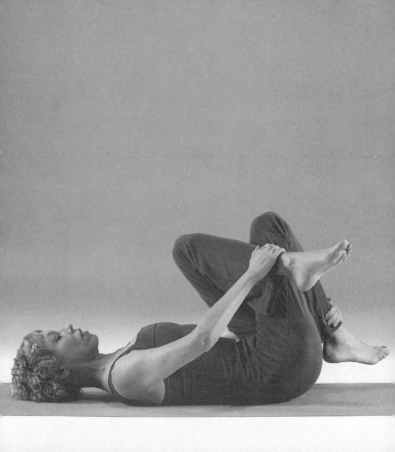

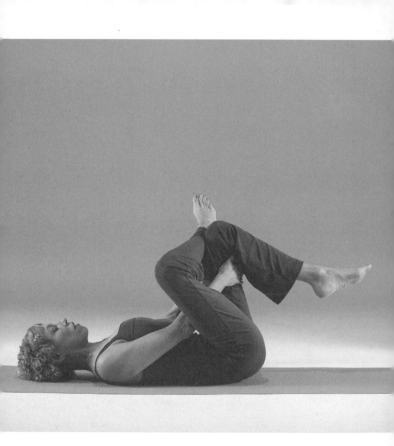

This is a slightly more advanced version of the previous exercise. It will help to release the hips.

Lying on your back with your legs bent, very gently cross the right ankle over the left knee. Make sure it's the ankle, and not the toes. Gently, keeping your knee open, bend the leg into the chest and feel a stretch on the bent leg. Remember, on all the stretches, you should only feel a stretch on the working leg. Hold for 30 seconds, change legs, and repeat four times.

Watchpoint

- With both the above exercises, if you feel a strain in your back – stop. This means you're working your legs too hard.

quadriceps stretch

Stand upright. Hold onto something if you feel you're losing your balance. Grasp one ankle and gently stretch the front of your thigh. Keep your knees in line (check in a mirror if you're not certain). Ensure that your stomach is in, and your tailbone dropped. You should be stretching from the hip flexor all the way down to the front of your thigh. Do not arch your back. Repeat four times, alternating legs. Hold for 30 seconds.

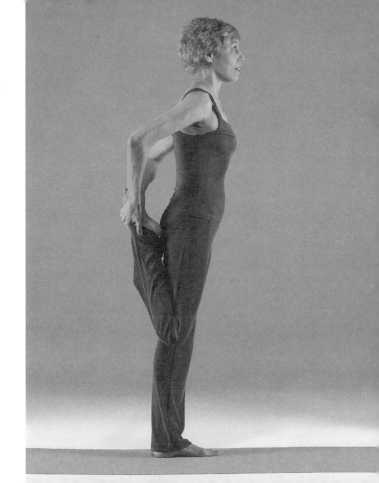

quadriceps stretch (advanced)

Kneel down on your right leg. Extend the left leg so that the knee is directly over the ankle. Gently pull your stomach in. Lean back slightly without arching your back. Hold for 30 seconds. Repeat four times, alternating legs.

Watchpoint

■ If this stretch causes pain in your knee or your back – stop.

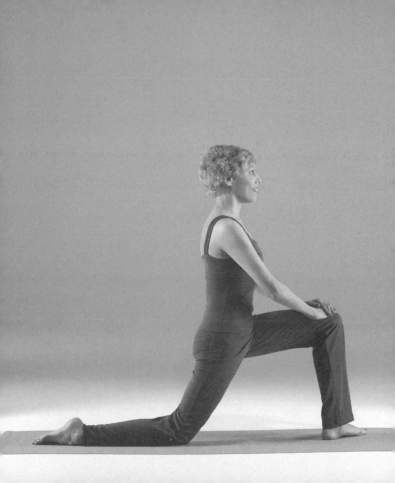

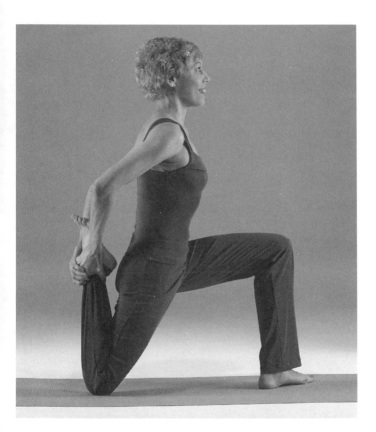

quadriceps stretch (advanced) 2

Assume the same position as the previous exercise. Holding your back foot, bend your knee and pull the foot towards your bottom. Keep your stomach in and don't arch your back. Hold for 30 seconds. Repeat four times, alternating legs.

Lying on your back, bend your knees into your chest. Place your hand behind the calf of the leg that you're working, and stretch the leg towards the ceiling. Keep your foot flexed. Hold for 30 seconds. Repeat four times, alternating legs.

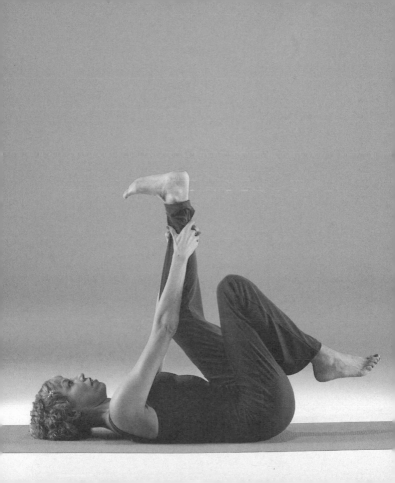

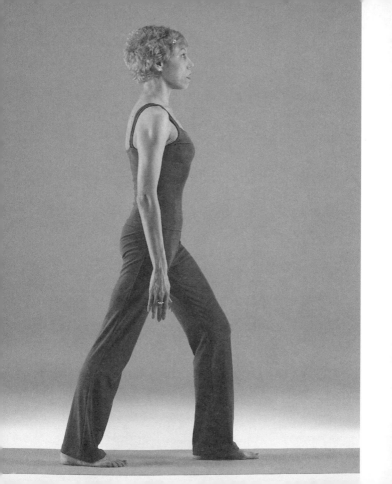

Stand up straight. Take a step forward with your right leg, bend the knee slightly, and feel the stretch down through the back leg. Keep your heel down on the back leg. Do not bounce. Hold for 30 seconds. Repeat four times, alternating legs.

Place your foot (gently flexed) on a chair and extend your leg. Keep the standing leg slightly bent and your stomach in. Neck and shoulders are relaxed. Hips are level. Slide your hands down towards your foot. You should feel the stretch in the muscle between the knee and the hip. Hold for 30 seconds. Repeat four times, alternating legs.

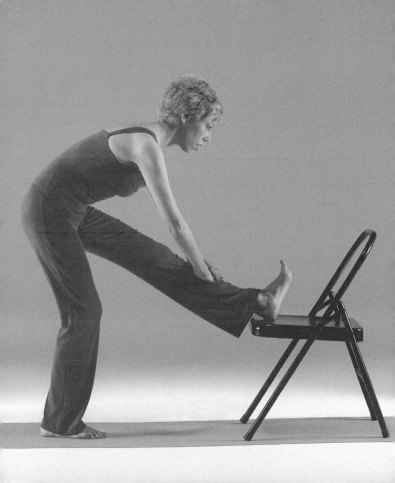

For this exercise, most people need to place a towel beneath the head. Lie on your mat or towel.

Start with both feet on the floor, making sure you have equal weight down through both feet. The arms are beside you and the pelvis is in the neutral position. Very gently bend your right knee into the chest. Grasp the back of your thigh with your left hand. Grasp the back of your calf with your right hand and gently unfold, straightening that leg with a flexed foot, and ease the leg towards you.

You'll know if you are doing it wrong if your bottom lifts. If this is impossible, instead of using your hands take a towel, place it around your calf and ease the leg towards you, keeping your neck and shoulders relaxed.

Do the right leg, then the left, and repeat, a minimum of twice on each side, holding for 30 seconds.

Watchpoint

- Don't pull on your leg so that your bottom leaves the floor, as your pelvis will twist. You want to flex the foot without overly tensing the feet, and gently straighten that knee. It is more important to get the knee straighter than to bring the leg closer to you.

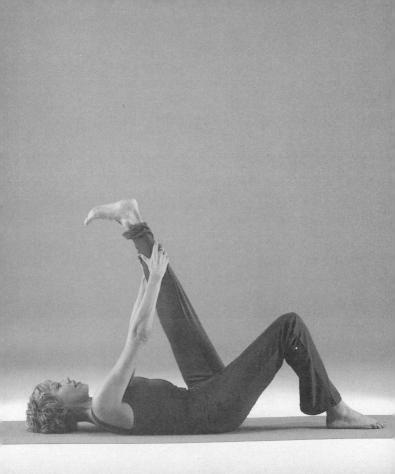

Sit on the floor with the soles of your feet together, stomach in. Hold onto both ankles. Gently drop your chin to your chest, relax your shoulders, and let your knees drop to the sides. Hold for 30 seconds. Repeat four times. If this is difficult, sit on a cushion to begin with.

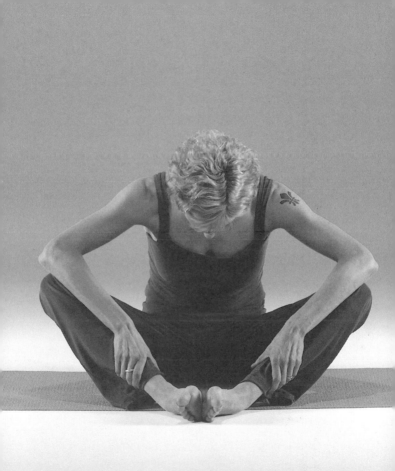

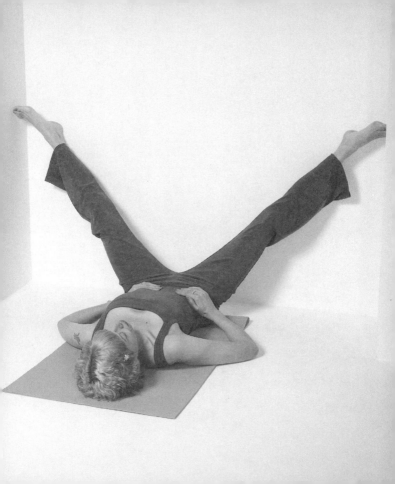

Lie on your back, with your legs up a wall. Let your legs fan out to the sides as far as is comfortable. Make sure your stomach is in, and your tailbone dropped. If you feel any pain in your knees, stop. Hold for 30 seconds. Bring your legs back together. Repeat four times.

This stretches the front of your thigh, the quadriceps
muscle.

Kneeling in a lunge position, holding on to a chair to
stabilize your weight, place one foot in front of you with the
knee bent. The knee should be directly above the ankle. If
the foot is behind the knee, you may strain your knee. You
can either have the toes pointing directly forward or at "10
to 2" (think of your foot as a clock hand). Do whatever feels
more comfortable for you. Due to the way in which your
lower leg is aligned, the position of comfort may vary.
Kneeling on the other leg, the foot behind you, very gently
pull your stomach in. Press your hips forward and feel a
stretch down the front of the thigh. At no point arch your
back. Your stomach is pulled in, your shoulders are relaxed
– imagine that someone has one hand on your stomach,
gently pushing your stomach in, and the other hand on your
bottom, which is being gently pushed forward to stabilize
your spine.

The harder version of this exercise is simply to take your
hands away from the chair, put them on your knee and take
slightly more of a lean back to get a stronger stretch, but
not at the expense of arching your back, straining your
knee, or letting your stomach protrude.

Repeat the exercise twice on each side, alternating legs.

Watchpoint

- Don't kneel on a hard floor as you may hurt your knee. With any exercises involving the knees, if you have any knee pain at any time, stop. Pain in the knee is contraindicated in any exercise.

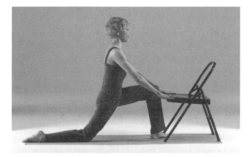

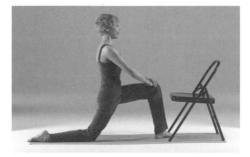

upper body exercises

In my experience as a Pilates teacher, all women want a beautiful upper back, gorgeous shoulders, and lovely arms and triceps. The following exercises will tone your back, arms, shoulders, and chest. The spine is the central structure of the body. Tight or weak back muscles will eventually lead to problems. Taking steps to strengthen one's back is insurance for the future. A strong back and center go hand in hand to present an upright and confident person.

You can do second sets when your body builds up to it and follow them with the stretches, which are absolutely essential after performing upper body work. Proper stretching will prevent you from having rounded shoulders and tight muscles.

One combination is press ups, dips, and then repeat. An alternative would be a tricep press, bicep curl, and then repeat.

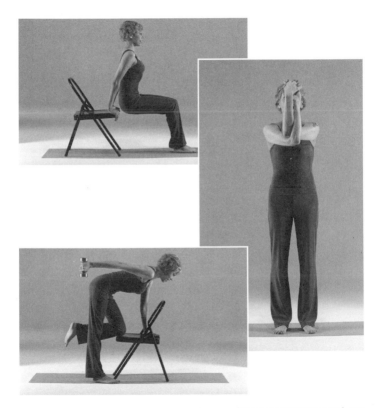

This exercise is a slight variation of a press-up, which I use a great deal in my studio.

On your hands and knees, make a square with the body. Again, it is better not to kneel on a hard surface – use a towel or an exercise mat. To begin, knees are under the hips; the hands are under the shoulders. Cross one hand over the other. The neck is in line. There is no arching the back, the stomach is pulled in. Do not lock the elbows.

In this position, very gently, working with your entire body, tip yourself slightly forward over the arms. This does not mean you should arch your back. It is very natural, when assuming the press-up position, to allow your head to drop. However, try to keep the head in a neutral position, neither forward nor backward.

Begin by doing six repetitions with the right hand on top, then the left. Work up to a set of 10 or 12 with each hand on top. Very gently breathe in as you bend the arms, bringing the chest down. Breathe out as you push away.

If it is possible, do the press-ups in front of a mirror. When you press down, your head should not lower and your chin should not stick out. When you start this exercise you will feel your weight rocking slightly forwards and backwards. Try to stabilize the weight over the arms so that you get the most strengthening through the upper back, the shoulders, the triceps and biceps muscles in the arms. You will be both strengthening and toning. This will not only result in a great-looking upper body, but you will be generating some upper-body strength as well. If you can't easily open your own bottle of champagne, then you have a problem.

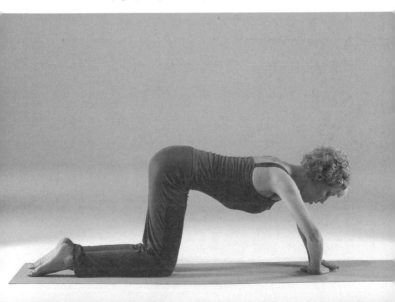

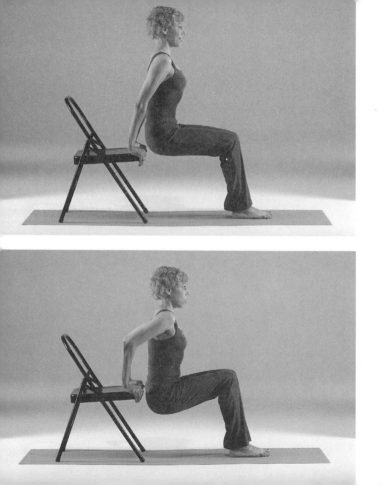

Most women find dips difficult to start with because of the
lack of strength in the backs of their arms.

Using a chair placed against a wall for support, have your
hands wide enough so that your shoulders don't feel
pinched together. Fingers are facing forward. Make sure in
this position that your knees are over your ankles. If they're
not you'll be using your thighs as opposed to the backs of
your arms. As you breathe in, you bend; as you breathe out,
you straighten.

Make sure as you do the dips that you're sliding your
bottom down the edge of the chair and that you're not
sliding forward, as the body will automatically prefer to do,
and taking the strain in the front of the thighs.

You might only be able to start with eight repetitions; gently
build up to 25.

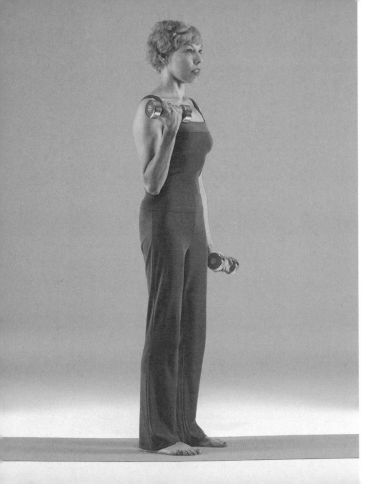

Holding a four-pound/two-kilo weight in each hand, breathe in and bend your arm up to shoulder level. Breathe out and straighten to waist level. Try not to rock as you do this. Repeat 10 to 15 times with alternate arms.

Using a firm chair, make a square with your body. Place
your left hand and knee on the chair, keeping your right leg
straight on the ground. Keep your neck in line with the rest
of your body. Holding the hand weight, lift your right arm up
as high as you can, keeping the elbow bent at a right angle,
without twisting the body. Exhale as you straighten the arm
behind you. Pause. Bend your arm back again. Repeat
10–15 times on each arm. You may do a second set.

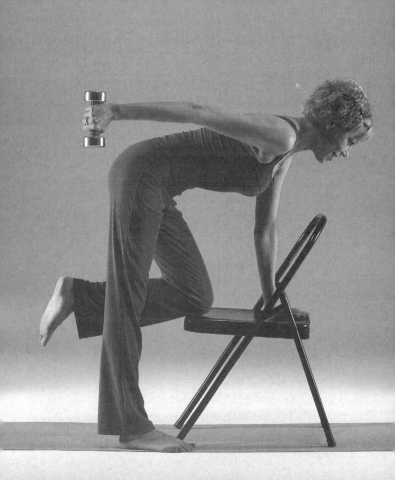

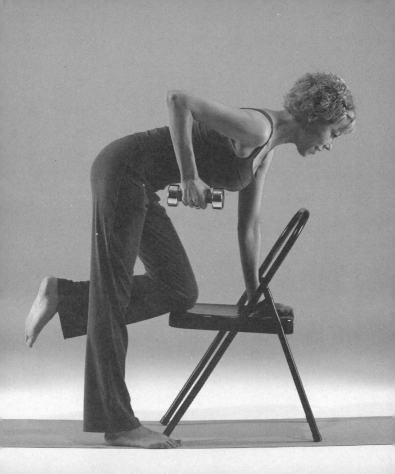

Assume the same position as in the previous exercise. (All the same rules apply.) This time you're using your arm to pull up and down. As you "pull" – feel your lats doing all the work – imagine you're pulling up weeds. Repeat 10–15 times on each arm. Do a second set if you wish.

Watchpoint

■ Do not use your shoulders to do the work in this exercise.

This stretch can be done seated or standing. Cross one arm over the other and clasp your hands together. Gently push your elbows to the ceiling and feel your shoulders stretching. As you press your arms up, try to keep your shoulders down. Keep your elbows in line with your shoulders. Hold for 10 seconds and then relax. Repeat four times, alternating arms.

Watchpoint

- If you feel any cramp or discomfort in your shoulders or arms, you are not yet flexible enough to do this.

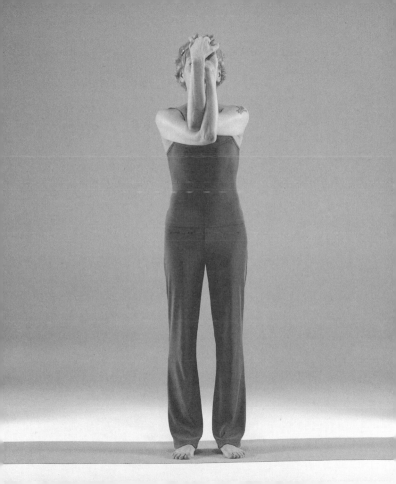

arm exercises

The following arm exercises are done lying on your back.
You should do them after your upper body work. They will
help you to keep your shoulders flexible. Place a towel
under your head if it feels more comfortable.

In all of these exercises remember to keep your back in a
neutral position: don't let your ribs lift. Keep your feet hip-
width apart, knees bent, with no tension in the lower back.

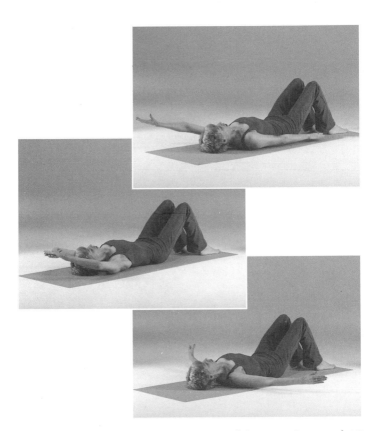

Lying on your back, raise your arms above your chest.
Imagine you're a tulip, and as you breathe out, your arms
gently open. As you breathe in, bring your arms back
together. Keep the curve in the elbows. Repeat 10 times,
opening and closing.

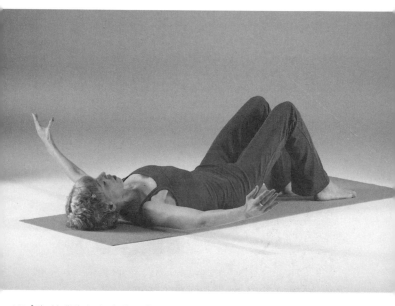

Start in the same position as above. Hold your arms over your chest. The palms face the wall in front of you. Keep your shoulders relaxed. As you breathe out, simultaneously one arm goes down in front of you and one behind you. Breathe in as you reverse the arms. Imagine you're doing the backstroke. Repeat 20 times, 10 on each side.

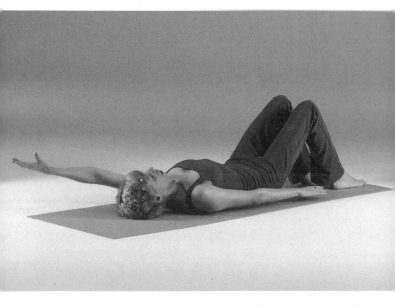

Assume the same position as in the previous exercise.
Place one hand gently over the other, so that you're making
a diamond shape with your elbows. As you breathe out,
take your arms as far back to the floor, past your ears, as
you can without your back lifting. Repeat 10 times,
alternating the hand on top.

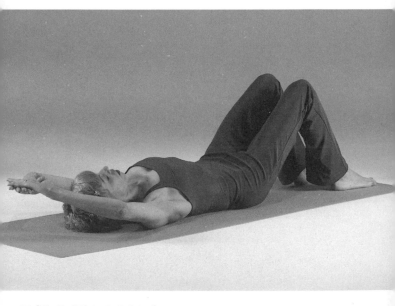

Assume the same position as in the Arms Opening
exercise on page 168. With your arms stretched up above
you, breathe out and make a circle, so that your hands
touch the floor all the way behind you. Bring your arms
back and stretch towards your hips. Repeat 10 circles
one way and 10 going the other.

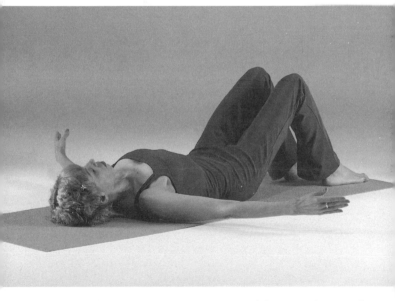

This is a great way to relax at the end of any program, but if you have any back pain don't do this.

Lean your back against a wall. Remember to always keep the knees bent, otherwise you risk straining your back.

Breathe out, and very slowly drop your chin to your chest. It helps if you count as you do this. Start to roll your back down, as gently as you can. By the time you get to a count of eight, your shoulders should roll off the wall. If your legs start to shake, bend your knees a bit more. Roll down as far as you feel comfortable and count for 10–20 seconds. Your arms should now be hanging loosely by your side like a puppet's. Gently move your head from side to side. Pause, and try to roll up, very slowly. Repeat four times (twice down, twice up).

Watchpoint

- If you've got low blood pressure don't do this, or you might feel faint.

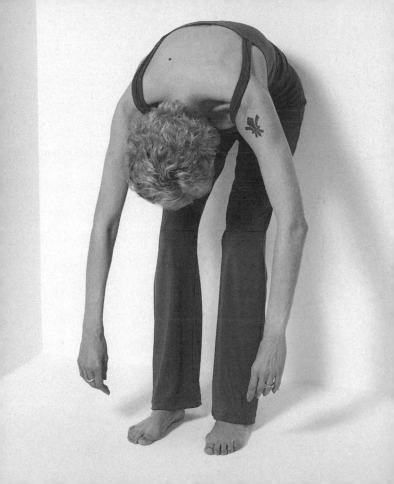

Lifestyles can create polarization. In other words, we may go from "living" at the gym to a total abstinence from any form of exercise, the most common reason being lack of time. I have tried to address this problem by weaving these exercises throughout a busy day, making it easier to implement movement during your free time.

specific programs

morning energizer

Sleep is supposed to restore us; it is the time when the body regenerates itself. Despite its obviously therapeutic uses, some people don't sleep terribly well. They may have disturbed slumber or they lie in uncomfortable positions.

Often people wake up feeling lethargic, tight, and tense. These exercises focus on limbering and release, and will enable you to start your day in a positive frame of mind. Doing these gentle mobilizing exercises early in the day will reconstruct some of the body's internal alignment. This group of six exercises will wake you up, stimulate you, and get your joints moving. They will also initiate the feeling of alignment – of standing up straight, feeling balanced and positive.

Concentrating on limbering and release, this 10-minute program of morning stretches focuses on releasing the lower spine and hips and gently loosening the upper body. The spine, the upper and lower back, and the muscles in the backs of your legs, the hamstrings, will be released. One movement, based on a classic Pilates exercise, opens up your spine and releases through your discs. Hip rotations will lubricate your hips. The arm exercises will open your shoulder girdle and start getting you to focus on breathing. Finally, there is a side stretch done with a towel to generally stretch and open up. The Morning Energizer should make you feel physical liberation and a spiritual awakening.

In all the exercises that involve lying on the floor, it is recommended that you use an exercise mat, but a large bath towel will do. Don't do these exercises on a wooden floor with only a towel. A bath towel placed on a carpet should give enough support to your spine.

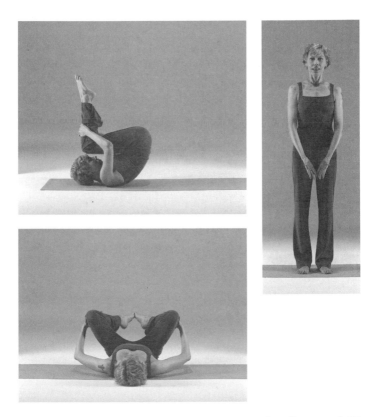

This exercise can be difficult; work your way into it. Sit holding on to your shins. From the photograph, you can see that I'm curled up like a ball. As you breathe out you roll backwards, and as you breathe in you roll up to a seated position.

Many people don't have a lot of flexibility in the spine, so you might have a problem in getting back up. If this is the case, come back up normally and start the roll again.

Try to keep the heels close to your bottom all the way through, and relax your shoulders. As you breathe out and roll back, the stomach pulls in. Do not roll too high up on the neck. All the exercises are done approximately 10 times. Rolling Up Like a Ball is the exercise I do first when I exercise.

Watchpoint

- Don't roll too far back onto your neck.

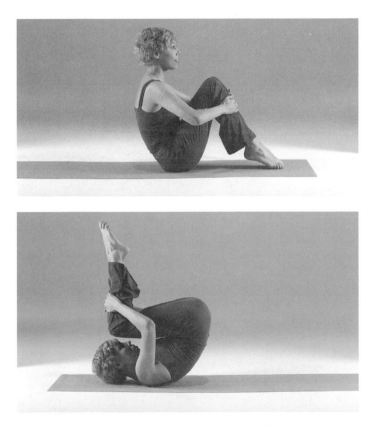

As we get older the hips get tighter, and there is less articulation in the hip socket.

Lie on a large towel or an exercise mat. Keep the feet together and hold on just below the knees. If you feel uncomfortable, put a towel behind your head. The body should not move, the head is resting.

Holding on below the knees, toes together, you rotate your hips 10 times in one direction and 10 times in the other, to lubricate your hips.

Keeping the toes together, start with the knees apart.

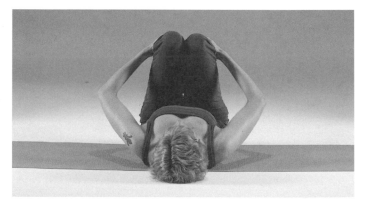

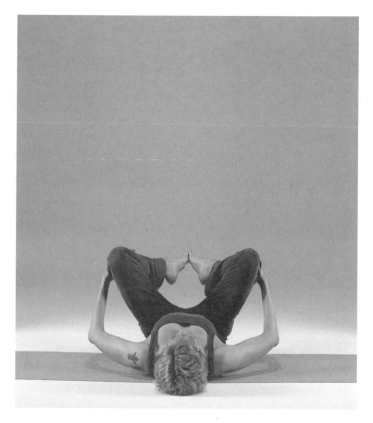

As you breathe normally, they come into the chest, then they open and come around. It doesn't matter in which direction you go. This exercise will also help to warm your lumbar spine and the entire pelvis area. You may feel a gentle stretch in your inside thighs if they're tight. Don't force this feeling of stretch. Just feel the mobilization. You're getting blood to flow through your hips and releasing

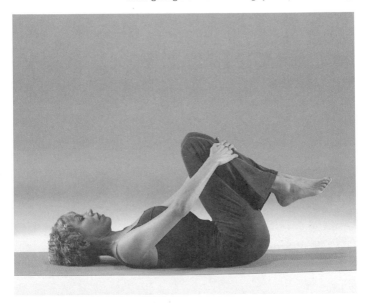

tension through your pelvis. Don't have the legs too far away from you. Keep the knees over the hips. Your legs do not hang off your body. Your tailbone is heavy and supported by the mat or towel at all times.

Watchpoint

■ Hold on to your shins and thighs, never the knees.

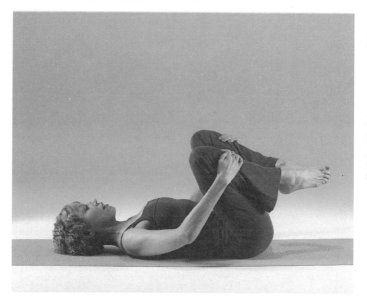

Lie on your back with a towel behind your head and flex
your feet – your toes pointing up towards your knees. Hold
your hands, fingers entwined. As you breathe in, the elbows
bend so the hands almost touch the crown of the head.

As you breathe out, stretch your arms as far away from you
as you can, flex your feet and stretch. Breathe in, bend your
elbows, relax, breathe out, and stretch. You'll feel this stretch
in the back of your legs, your hamstrings, your calf muscles,
feet, and shoulders. You may feel a stomach stretch as well.

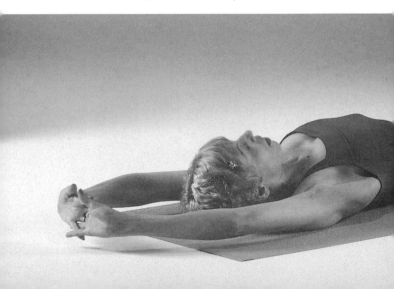

Do approximately 10 repetitions.

You can either do this exercise with the hands crossed or
the fingers interlaced. Breathe in, breathe out, and stretch.
As you breathe out and stretch, the shoulders shrug up
towards the ears. As you breathe in, relax the shoulders,
and let them drop. The hands come towards the crown of
your head or forehead, the legs relax. As you breathe out,
the fingers and hands stretch away, the shoulders lift, the
flexed feet stretch towards the other end of the room. The
body is stretched and energized.

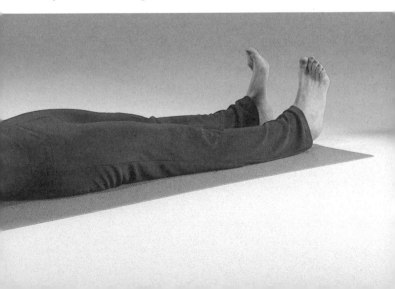

This and the following exercise are about postural awareness. At this point do not stand on a towel unless you feel very secure. This exercise is better done with bare feet, so you can feel the contact with the floor.

Stand with your feet hip-width apart. Relax your feet. Make sure the weight is evenly placed over your feet, try not to sink either forward or backward. The toes are relaxed and lengthened as if they're softening into sand. When you're standing upright the stomach is gently pulled in, the tailbone drops, the pelvis is in neutral. You're not gripping your hamstrings or the back or front of your legs.

Your arms should be naturally relaxed at your side. They don't hang behind you, they gently soften, as if your middle finger is stretching down the outside of your thigh, lengthening away. In this position the hands are just in front of you. The shoulders are relaxed and the head is in a neutral position. Don't let your head drop forward or back. Let it sit on top of your shoulders. Use visualization techniques and think of your head as a blossom sitting on the stem of a plant. The head is just softly there. The knees are released.

Begin by breathing out. As you do so, one arm reaches to the ceiling, and the other arm gently reaches to the wall behind you without any shift in the feet, the pelvis, the upper back, or the neck. If you're feeling that shift you are

taking the movement too far for your initial flexibility. This
exercise can be done either 10 times, five on each side, or
20, which is 10 on each side, alternating the arms.

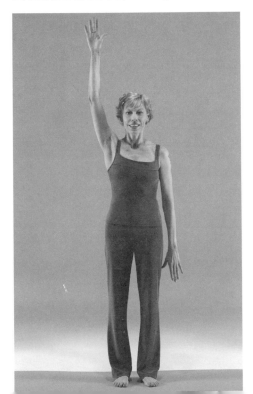

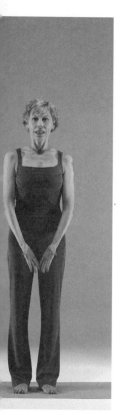

This exercise targets the same area as the previous one. Start with the same postural alignment, no gripping of the feet, no tensing of the buttocks – everything is relaxed and calm. Straighten both your arms and bring them in front of you with the tips of the little fingers touching.

As you breathe out, take a slice and reach to the corners of the room. The arms stay straight all the way through. Breathe in, breathe out, then slice, reaching for the corners of the room.

Watchpoint

- With any of the arm exercises, at no point do you lock your elbows. The joints are in line: the shoulders, the elbows, the wrist, all the fingers – don't break at the wrist.

After you've done this second exercise 10 times you may do a few on the diagonal. You slice, gently twist and the head follows. You will feel a gentle stretch across the chest and some stretching through the shoulders.

These exercises are also about coordination. In the first exercise both arms work rhythmically, alternating. In the second exercise you want both arms to start and end at the same point. You don't want one arm to begin before the other.

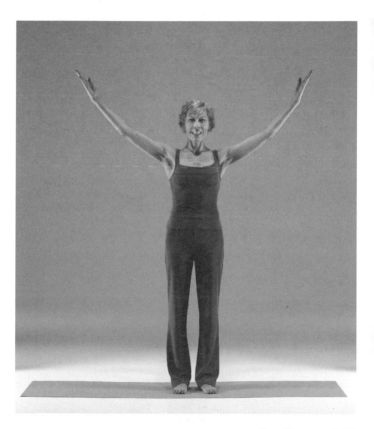

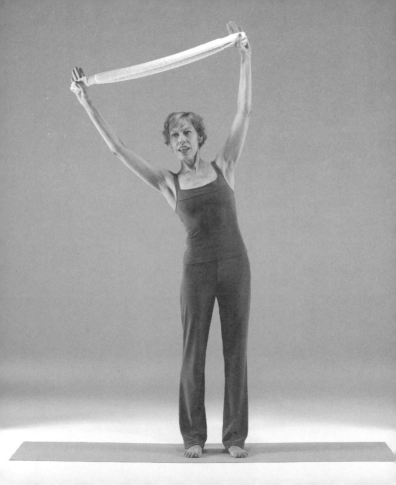

Stand in the same position, holding a folded hand towel nice and wide between your arms. Breathe out, stretch to one side. Breathe in, straighten up, and breathe out to stretch to the other side. Don't lift your shoulders up to your ears, and stretch only as far as you can without shortening on the underneath side.

Your weight should be evenly balanced over both feet. You'll know you've gone too far if you feel one foot coming off the floor. The weight is over the second toe, as in all of the standing exercises. Hips don't move very much because it is a waist-energizing stretch. Breathe out as you take the stretch, breathe into the center, and breathe out as you change.

Do approximately 10 repetitions on each side.

The waist stretch is related to core strength. You engage your abdominals to stabilize your pelvis and your spine during a gentle waist stretch; the body does not collapse from side to side.

Watchpoint

- Keep the weight evenly distributed over both feet for the duration of the exercise and don't allow yourself to tip from one side to the other.

With these exercises you will maximize posture and energy levels in environmentally unfriendly conditions. You will learn to sit and stand correctly throughout the day. New habits will form and, once learned, will be hard to break. Your body will feel comfortable and well balanced, freeing you to be mentally alert.

Generally, people sit badly. They sink into their hips when they sit down. Most people are not as active as they should be because of the restrictions in their daily lives. These exercises will take you back to basics, re-creating the way you sit. The emphasis in these exercises is not on complicated movement but on visualization.

You are sitting at your desk, with your chair at the right level, with your feet grounded through the floor, and equal pressure down through both feet. Your lower back is supported in the chair, the upper back floating above with no tension. A shoulder stretch has also been included, which will release tense shoulders. You then breathe into your stomach and, on the exhale, you contract your stomach into the back of the chair, concentrating on feeling that movement of internal support as you grow taller and more confident.

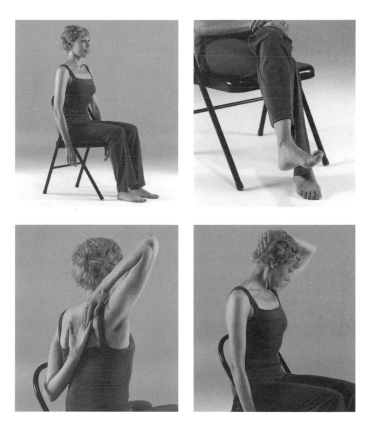

Sit with your back supported by a chair. Your tailbone is heavy, both feet are evenly placed on the floor. You are in contact from your center directly down through your feet into the floor. You're going to channel your energies from your center out through the crown of your head. Your shoulders are relaxed, your arms are relaxed because your middle back is supported. Your tailbone will drop and your abdominals will naturally pull back towards your spine. Again, try to think of your head sitting naturally on top of your shoulders, not pushing forward and not pushing back.

Watchpoint

- If you force your shoulders back and your lower back arches away from the chair, you know your shoulders are still too rounded for you to maintain this position and be anatomically correct.

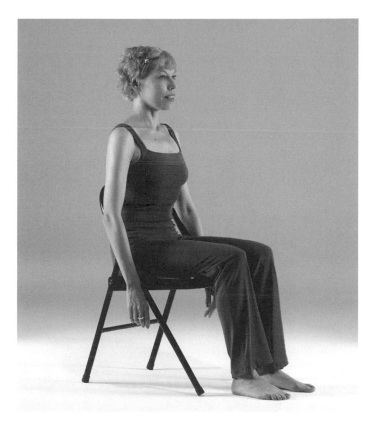

Starting with this basic seated position, place your fingers on your lower abdominals, the space between your pubic bone and your navel. As you breathe in the stomach gently expands, filling with oxygen. As you breathe out the stomach pulls away from your fingers and settles back into the chair, your navel pulls away from your fingers and you feel the energy going in to support the lower back. Repeat 10 times.

You can either have your fingers on your abdomen in the same place as the previous exercise or allow your arms to hang naturally beside you. As you breathe in your abdomen gently softens or expands into your fingers, as you breathe out you very gently let one foot float off the floor, feeling the connection of the navel to the spine. Place the foot down, make sure you have even pressure through both feet again, and change legs. The coordination is important. Start off foot lifts very slowly; eventually you will be able to do them faster so the interchange emanates from a stable pelvis and a strong abdomen.

Initially the change from one leg to the other might feel unstable as you don't have the core strength to coordinate alternate leg lifts automatically. The feet should float off the floor. Do 10 lifts with each leg, alternating each time.

Watchpoint

- If you lift your feet too high, you will feel your pelvis sink back into the chair and you'll lose that postural alignment. Your tailbone will tuck underneath and your back will curl.

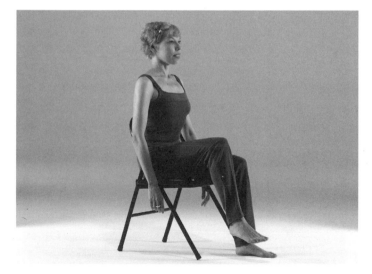

This exercise will relax your ankle, calf, and foot, and it will give you a conscious feeling of the connection between your body and the earth.

Slip your shoes off, cross one knee over the other and gently circle your ankle very slowly, so that you take six seconds to circle the ankle in one direction, approximately six to eight times. Change directions and repeat, then do the same thing with the other ankle.

Watchpoint

■ Try to keep your toes relaxed, don't grip with your toes. Do not move the bones in your lower leg (the tibia and fibula). Think of your ankle bones as pebbles that you're gently shaking. As you're circling the ankle, the pebbles are lubricating and relaxing. If you tense your foot and lower leg, this won't happen. Your ankle and calf will feel warmer after this exercise, if completed slowly and rhythmically.

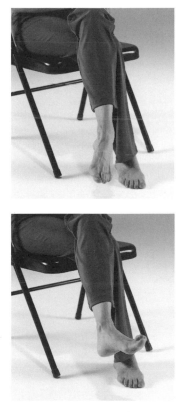

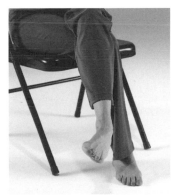

Seated in your chair, all the previous rules apply: stomach pulled in, tailbone dropped, both feet evenly balanced on the floor. Think of your energy evenly placed down through both feet. Very gently, take your right hand and place it on your left shoulder blade, palm facing down. Take your other hand and try to reach and connect your fingers behind you. If you can't do this initially, don't worry, aim to do it eventually. Without arching your back or sticking your chest out, gently open out the right or the left top arm to stretch. Keep the neck long. Do the other side, then approximately five times on each side, alternating sides.

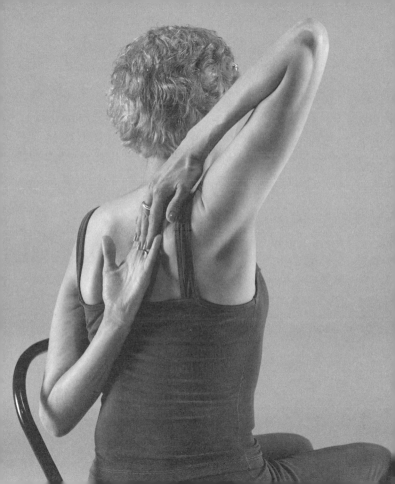

This neck stretch should not be done more than four times.

Sitting in your chair, gently place the palm of your hand not on your neck, but behind the crown of your head.

Sit with your feet comfortably apart, drop your chin towards your chest without leaning forward, look at your big toe and gently press your head against your hand; feel the neck stretching. Hold for 20 seconds. Relax, do the stretch on the left and once more on either side.

Watchpoint

- The middle back should be supported, the tailbone dropped; don't let the chin go forward.

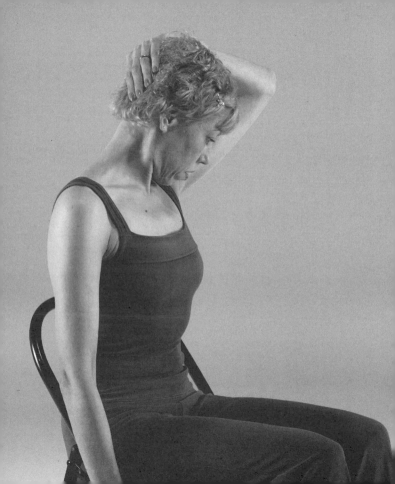

midday break

The human mind and body don't function at their best after working for eight consecutive hours. You need to have a space or break in your working day, whether it's a brisk walk or reading a newspaper. A change of environment – physical or mental – will recharge your batteries. Your mind and body will be clearer and you'll feel less sluggish in your working environment.

An active aerobic break combined with stretches and body-releasing exercises makes a lunch break a good time to rejuvenate and recharge. "Aerobic" is a very general term that can indicate anything from climbing the stairs to taking a short walk.

This program is a restart and refocus. It involves a lot of stretching.

It will address the areas that are tight from sitting and working, and will be especially helpful for those who work in front of a computer screen.

You will stand up and do some very simple foot exercises, such as grasping the floor with your toes and releasing, followed by calf stretches, a few shoulder stretches, and a cat stretch. There is also a stretch in which you stand in the doorway and release your shoulders.

This focuses the energy away from areas of work-induced tightness so you can feel relaxed and liberated when you lunch. You can then enjoy your lunch break, as you will have rid yourself of work-related muscular stress.

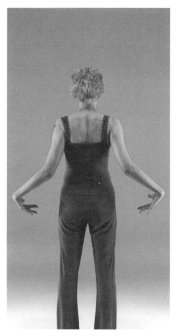

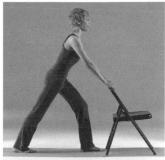

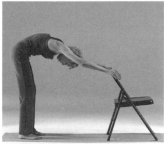

Doming is better done with bare feet. Very gently lift your foot so that you're just resting on your heel. As you place your foot on the ground, spread your toes and try to separate them. Ideally they will all spread and separate at the same time. (Imagine doming with your hand: you lift and separate your fingers as you place them down.)

Holding your toes down, you draw up the arch underneath your foot, without gripping your toes. Relax. As you flex onto the heel and spread the toes, imagine having chewing gum under the ball of your foot. You draw your toes up – without gripping the floor – and relax. In the beginning you might get cramp in your foot. Do 10 repetitions with each foot.

Watchpoint

- Do not let your toes become "clawed."

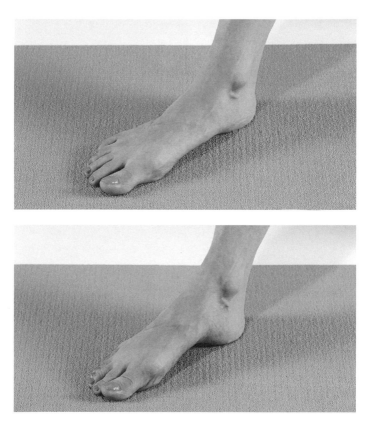

Again, this exercise is done without shoes. Using your
office desk or chair, do a very simple calf stretch.
Shoulders are down, the stomach is in, the tailbone
dropped. Don't arch your back or stick out your ribs. Keep
your shoulders down and the head floating on top of your
body. Have both feet hip-width apart, take a step forward
with one leg and feel a stretch down the back of the other,
the heel touching the floor. Hold for 30 seconds, then do
the other leg. Repeat again.

Watchpoint

- Keep the stomach in, the tailbone dropped.

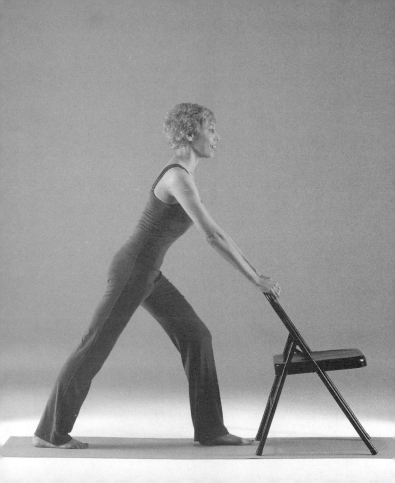

This exercise will open up your shoulders. It can be done seated in an office chair, but the preferred position is against a door frame or wall.

Lean with your knees bent and middle back against the wall, and slide down, keeping the knees bent. Your weight is placed evenly over the feet, which are not tense. Your middle back and the space between your shoulder blades touch the wall for support. Do not push your head back as you will feel your middle back and shoulder blades come off the wall.

Breathing normally, gently place your hands on your shoulders. This exercise consists of four movements: circle arms forward, trying to get the elbows to touch, lift up towards the ears, circle as far back as you can without any of your middle back coming off the wall. When you have completed the movement, you then circle the other way. Back, up, around and down. Do 10 repetitions in each direction.

Watchpoint

■ Keep your middle back and the space between the shoulder blades on the wall.

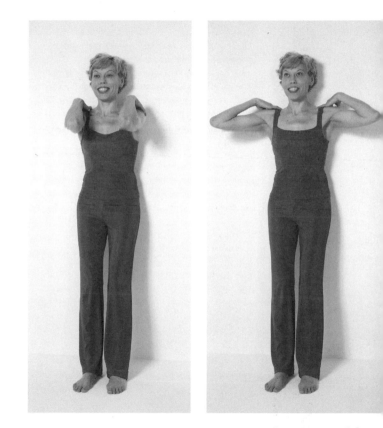

These two exercises will help those with stiff hands or people suffering from repetitive strain injury.

Sit or stand with your shoulders relaxed. Stretch your hands very gently and bring each finger to the thumb, beginning with the little finger. Stretch each of your fingers as much as you can.

This next exercise can be done either with your hands in front of you or behind you. The movement is exactly the same as above, but in this instance you circle the wrist. Think of Balinese dancers. This exercise also works on coordination.

Watchpoint
- Keep the shoulders and elbows relaxed.

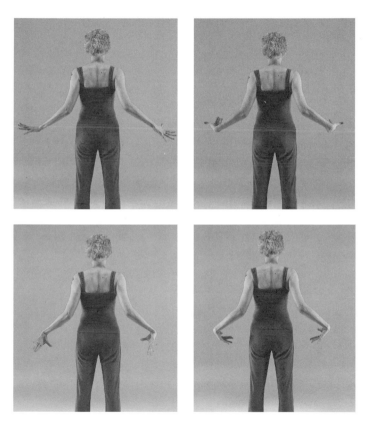

Using an office desk or chair, this exercise will release your lower back and stretch out your shoulders. Take your shoes off unless you're in flat shoes. Do not do this exercise in heels.

Stand as far away from your desk as you can while still resting your palms on the desk. Bend your knees slightly and keep them bent. Weight goes down evenly through both feet.

Breathe out, curl your chin into your chest, your stomach into your spine. Stretch out your lower back. This will counteract the effects of being seated for long periods of time, and get the blood flowing as you open your spine.

As you breathe in, press your chest down; your bottom goes up and the head gently lengthens back.

Watchpoint

- If you feel the neck crunching or your vocal cords contracting you've taken your head too far back. There should be no discomfort in your neck.

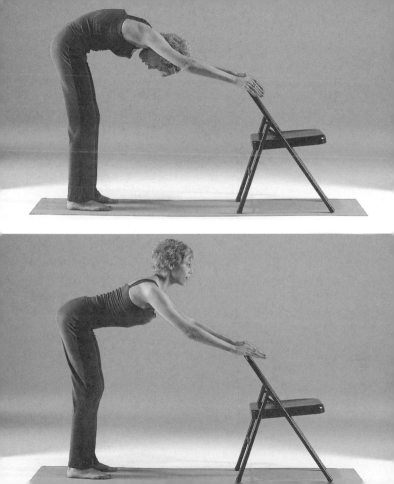

Again, stand as far away from your desk as you can with your palms resting on it. Bend your knees slightly and keep them bent. Weight goes down evenly through both feet.

For this shoulder stretch keep the ears between the arms. Holding on to the desk, press your chest down and stretch your arms to give your shoulders, neck, and upper arms a good stretch. Don't worry if you feel a little ache in your upper arms because it is "referred pain" from stretching out your upper back.

Watchpoint

- Keep knees bent and head between the arms.

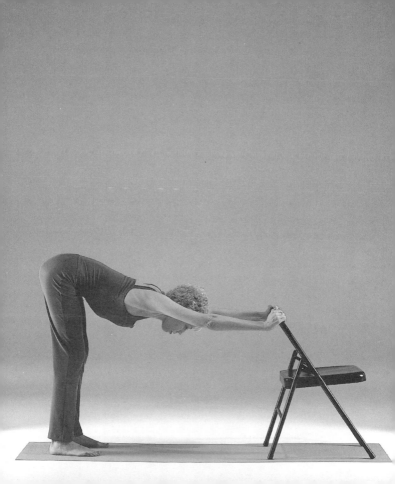

For those of you who have any condition that affects muscles and joints, my Body Maintenance program is a superb tool to use as you begin the journey towards helping and even reversing your condition.

remedial exercises

**I absolutely believe everyone can and will improve,
and even overcome, their physical difficulties with a
safe and gentle group of exercises. You will be
amazed at the body's ability to respond and
rejuvenate, given the correct impetus. In this chapter
are some specific exercises you can do every day to
alleviate repetitive strain injury (carpal tunnel
syndrome), scoliosis, sciatica, or a bad back.**

Note: The few remedial exercises contained in this book for
each condition will not achieve the results possible in my
studio and from individually taught programs over an
extended period of time.

The back causes more problems than almost any other part of the body. The spinal column provides support to the entire body and is the center of all movement. The muscles in the back link the vertebrae of the spine to each other. It is not surprising, then, that if these muscles are weak or damaged through injury, all sorts of problems affecting alignment and stability may occur.

Muscular pain and stiffness in the joints can transpire for many different reasons, for example congenital conditions, injury, weak muscles, a slipped disc, etc. The shock-absorbing discs between the vertebrae may slip out of position and can damage the joints, leading to infections and degenerative problems. Pain varies depending on the cause of the problem and the person.

Conventional treatment

Treatment may include anti-inflammatory drugs and painkillers, physiotherapy, and surgery. Back problems can be notoriously difficult to eliminate.

Body Maintenance method

Pilates-based exercises, as they focus on strengthening the muscles in the spine and abdomen, can be extremely beneficial for all sorts of back problems.

This 10-minute exercise program is based on the exercises that many of my clients who have had back injuries or who suffer from chronic back pain do first thing in the morning. When you wake up in the morning with a bad back, you tend to feel quite immobile, stiff, and uncomfortable. Your body doesn't want to move and you have difficulty even straightening up. This is a selection of six exercises to do in the morning between the time you get out of bed and go to work, which will strengthen and mobilize your lower back.

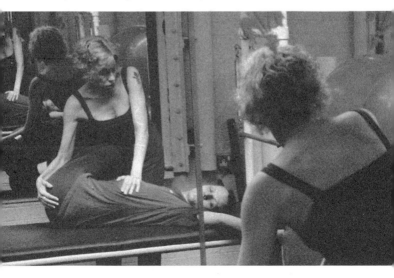

This is a basic pelvic tilt. Lie on a towel or mat. You may also need to place a small towel behind your head. The feet, hips, and knees are all parallel, hip-width apart; the tailbone is relaxed on the mat without feeling forced down. The shoulders are relaxed and the neck is long. The arms are softly beside you.

Without gripping your bottom, very gently tip your pelvis upwards as you breathe out, breathe in and lower. This is a low pelvic tilt. Don't lift higher than your waist. You are only lifting your lower back off the ground. It is important to exhale as you lift. Breathe in, keeping your neck long, and roll all the way down. Do approximately 10 repetitions.

Try to get that primary curve in your lower back working to warm up the lower back, bringing the blood supply into that area.

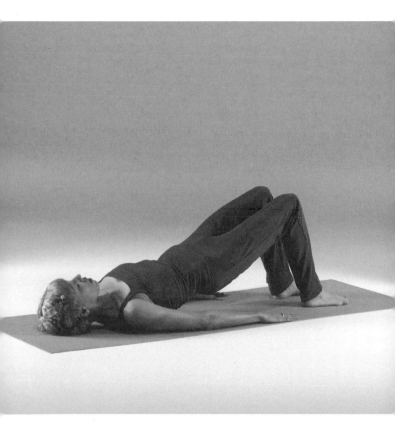

This is a passive stretch for the lower back and the hamstrings.

Lie in the same position as for the previous exercise. Very gently bend your right knee into your chest, holding on to the shin, below the kneecap. Have the elbows lifted to the side. You should not feel tension in your shoulders.

Breathe out and pull one knee into your chest, stretching the other leg along the floor and gently flexing both feet. You should feel a passive stretch going through the bent leg and buttock. You will also feel a hamstring and calf stretch going through the straight leg. Count: one, two, three, four. Then change sides. Do 10 repetitions altogether, alternating five on each leg.

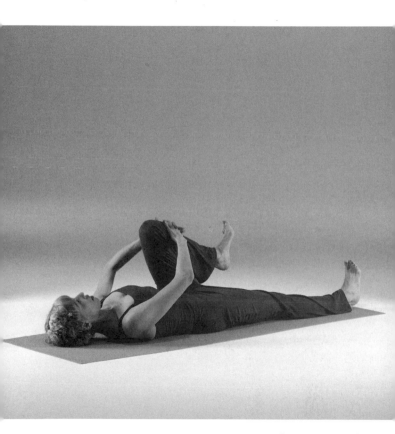

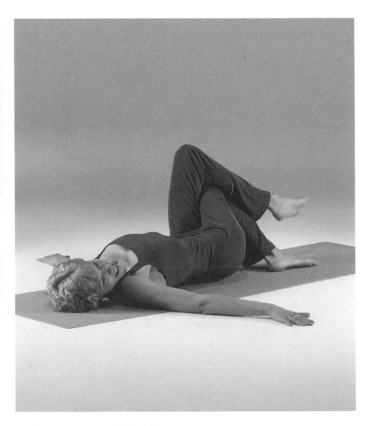

This mobilization exercise for the spine will warm up the back. It is a gentle stretch for the lower back and the hip. The stomach is the instigator of the movement. You are in exactly the same position as for the previous exercise, but this time you cross one leg over the other. It doesn't matter which leg you start with, but the other foot is firmly on the floor.

The arms are beside you, palms facing down below shoulder level. The stomach is the stabilizer in this exercise, and at no point does either shoulder blade leave the mat.

Breathe in, breathe out and take a gentle twist one way, looking away from the direction you are twisting towards. Come back to the original position. Breathe in from the center, and breathe out as you twist in the opposite direction.

You'll know if you've gone too far, as your stomach will protrude and your shoulders will leave the mat. If it's too hard for you to move your head and look in the opposite direction due to coordination problems, start by looking directly up while you familiarize yourself with the exercise. When you're comfortable you can begin turning the head.

Do 10 twists with one leg on top, then 10 twists with the other.

If you have a bad back, it is very likely that your buttock
muscles and hamstrings will be tight. Sit on the floor, or
lean against a wall.

Stretch your left leg out in front of you. Cross your right foot
over your left knee, keeping your right hand on the floor.
Hold on to your right knee with your left hand, as you gently
ease that knee into your chest. Then rotate your body
around to the right. The left leg in front of you is parallel to
the floor. Keep your foot to the ceiling and your shoulders
relaxed. Don't let your foot roll out of line with the knee.
Feel the stretch through your buttock.

Repeat four times, each time alternating legs and the
direction you turn. Hold each stretch for 30 seconds.

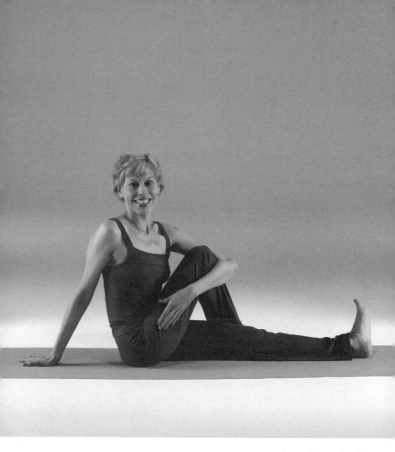

Lie face down, stomach on the floor. Relax your head to the side. Gently breathe in, and feel your stomach drop to the floor. Breathe out and pull your stomach into your spine so that your tailbone drops. Don't grip your bottom or tense your shoulders. Eventually you will be able to get your fingers in between your stomach and the floor as you breathe out. Feel your stomach working and your back strengthening. Both hipbones stay on the floor. Repeat 10 times.

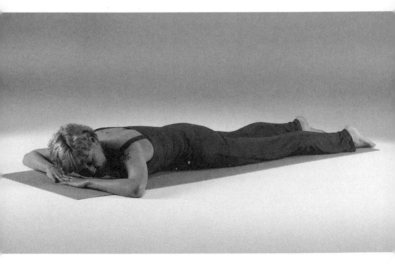

Roll over onto your back. Breathe in, then very gently
breathe out and, bending both knees to your chest, curl
your head towards your knees. Hold, breathe in, then
breathe out, and relax your head down, pulling your
stomach into your spine. This is a passive back and neck
stretch to stretch out your back. Do 10 repetitions.

Watchpoint

■ Don't tense your shoulders; keep your bottom on the floor.

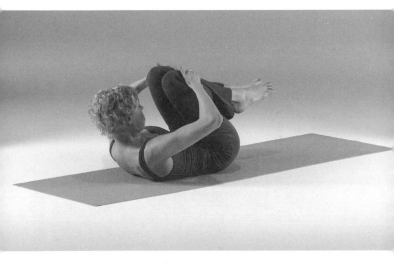

Sciatica is a radiating pain along the distribution of the sciatic nerve, which affects the buttocks and backs of the legs. It frequently causes pain in the lower back, or lumbago. In severe cases it may spread to the calf. The most common cause of sciatica is from a prolapsed intervertebral disc. This causes pressure on one or more of the nerve roots that originate in the lower part of the spinal cord and make up the sciatic nerve. Sciatica may also occur for a number of other reasons. For example, this condition may happen suddenly when a person is lifting something heavy. The amount of pain varies, depending on which nerve roots are affected, and ranges from mild discomfort to acute pain.

Conventional treatment

The first course of action is usually a few weeks of bed rest. Sometimes sufferers are prescribed a spinal support or corset. If there is no improvement, the next step may involve surgery in order to remove the compression of the disc on the nerve root.

Body Maintenance method

Pilates-based exercises can do much to alleviate this debilitating condition. Try the following exercises:

Lie on your stomach with your feet relaxed. Your arms
should be facing forwards and be just wider than your
shoulders, which are relaxed. Keep your neck "long" by
looking down. Keep looking down as you gently press your
hips and elbows into the floor and pull your stomach in.
Gently, lift your head up (keep it independent of the body),
focusing your eyes on the same point. Make sure you keep
your feet on the floor. Breathe in, and gently come down.
Feel your buttocks contract slightly. Do not contract them
too much – otherwise you're using your buttock muscles
and not the stomach. Engaging the abdominals helps to
strengthen your back and lift your body.

As you breathe out and lift, imagine that the crown of your
head is going forward towards the wall in front of you. Do
not lift your head towards the ceiling. Ideally, you want as
little pressure on the hands as possible. Relax your fingers
and feel your shoulder blades releasing. Relax down again.

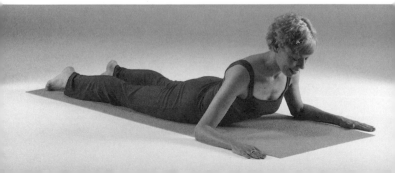

Stretch your left leg out in front of you. Cross your right foot
over your left knee, keeping your right hand on the floor.
Hold on to your right knee with your left hand, as you gently
ease that knee into your chest. Then rotate your body
around to the right. The left leg in front of you is parallel to
the floor. Keep your foot to the ceiling and your shoulders
relaxed. Don't let your foot roll out of line with the knee.
Feel the stretch through your buttock.

Repeat four times, each time alternating legs and the
direction you turn. Hold each stretch for 30 seconds.

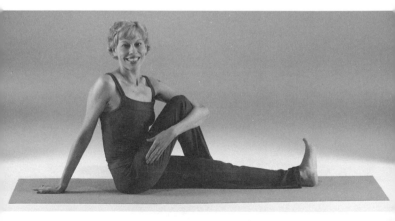

Lie face down, stomach on the floor. Relax your head to the side. Gently breathe in, and feel your stomach drop to the floor. Breathe out and pull your stomach into your spine so that your tailbone drops. Don't grip your bottom or tense your shoulders. Eventually you will be able to get your fingers in between your stomach and the floor as you breathe out. Feel your stomach working and your back strengthening. Both hipbones stay on the floor. Repeat 10 times.

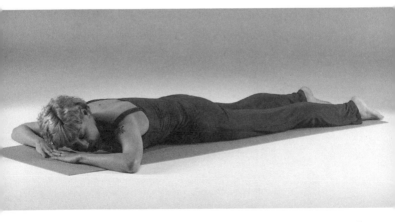

repetitive strain injury (carpal tunnel syndrome)

This is a common problem amongst people whose work involves some kind of repetitive action, such as typing at a keyboard all day or playing a musical instrument. There are various types of injury that can be sustained in the muscles, tendons, and ligaments in the hands and wrists from repetitive motions. The most common is the compression of the median nerve as it passes under the ligament that lies across the front of the wrist.

Symptoms appear after prolonged activity, and include tingling and weakness or numbness in the fingers and hands. Sufferers may also experience aching, burning, or shooting pains in the wrists and hands, which frequently spread to the forearms, neck, shoulders, upper back, and upper arms. These symptoms get progressively worse until the person is barely able to use his or her hands at all, as the weakness makes it almost impossible to grasp objects properly. In the most severe cases the fingers may also swell up.

Conventional treatment

Anti-inflammatory drugs, which may be prescribed to reduce the inflammation and swelling, aren't always effective. Painkillers can obviously help to relieve the pain, and wearing a splint can immobilize the wrist and alleviate discomfort.

Sufferers find that symptoms can come and go over the years. If the condition is not treated, the pain may become intolerable. Some people have to resort to surgery, which involves making an incision from the anterior of the wrist to the palm of the hand. The surgical effects are variable and symptoms may continue afterwards.

Body Maintenance method

I have seen many people make a good recovery using the specific exercises I have evolved to treat this condition. These exercises are very gentle. They are designed to strengthen the hands and wrists and should be practiced daily. As the hands and wrists get stronger and begin to regain proper mobility through exercise, the symptoms may disappear.

Holding onto your wrist with the other hand, make a fist with your hand. The wrist is in neutral. Gently lower your wrist down halfway, then bring it back to neutral again. Think of this as a resistance exercise. Imagine you're resisting very slowly. You can also do this with your hand facing up. Repeat 10 times.

You can do this using a small weight too (e.g., a can of beans), but not if you feel any pain.

wrist circles

Holding onto your wrist with the other hand, circle the wrist slowly one way, and then the other. Repeat 10 times, then change hands.

Watchpoint

- If you're doing these exercises correctly your hands and wrists will feel warmer.

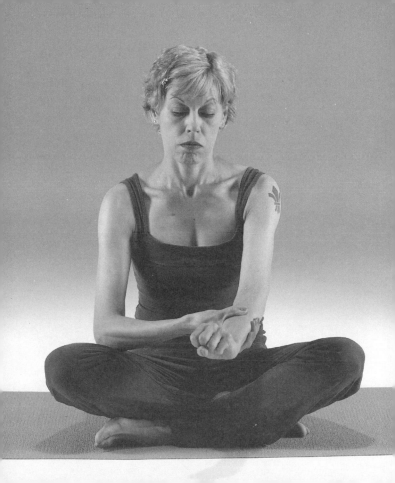

Place your hands so that the tips of the fingers and thumbs are touching. Imagine you're holding a soft ball. Press and resist your fingers – your hands don't close. Keep your shoulders relaxed and hands level with your chest. Relax and repeat 10 times.

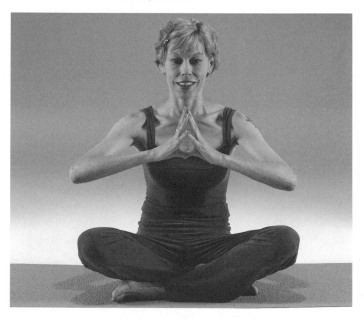

Using a chair, place your hands on the seat, fingers towards you. Keep your elbows unlocked and gently lean your wrists into the chair. Don't press with your whole weight. Repeat four times. Shake your hands afterwards. Remember: don't lean too hard into the stretch.

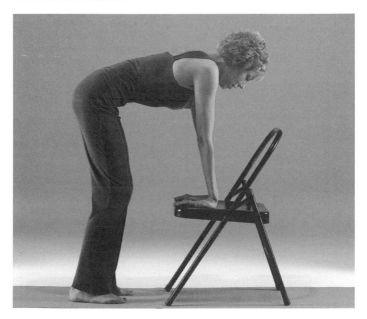

scoliosis

Scoliosis is an extremely distressing condition that generates an S-shaped curvature of the spine. This is caused by a twist in the spine, which leads to the vertebrae becoming compressed and tilting to one side. In time this pressure can bring about fused vertebrae. Symptoms vary depending on the degree of the twist. There is generally a great deal of distress as the body struggles to accommodate this spinal imbalance, which forces the surrounding muscles into painful contortions.

Mild scoliosis may be barely noticeable, but in severe cases it leads to the formation of an unsightly hump and causes constant stooping, as the person is unable to stand upright. Scoliosis tends to first appear in adolescence and from then on, unless it is corrected while the body is still young and malleable, gets progressively worse.

Conventional treatment

Treatment is usually very difficult. The most likely options for the scoliosis sufferer range from physiotherapy to surgical intervention. There are now several complex types of operations to try to correct it, or at least prevent the condition from worsening. However, these are not always successful.

Body Maintenance method

I have devised a number of exercises designed to build up the weak muscles in the back and uncurl the spine, and have been witness to some remarkable changes.

This is very similar to a basic pelvic tilt exercise, the only difference being that you cross one leg over the other.

Lie on your back, with one leg crossed over the other. Arms should be relaxed at your sides, with palms facing the floor. Allow your back to keep its natural arch. Don't press it down – keep it in a neutral spine position. Try very hard not to tense your buttock muscles.

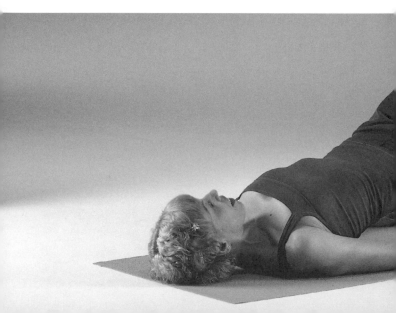

As you breathe out, gently tuck your pelvis under and curl your spine off the floor – through the lower back and into the middle back – until you're at the level just below your lower shoulder blades. Breathe in, keeping your neck long, and then very slowly roll down through the top of your spine, exhaling all the way down. Move one vertebra at a time, lowering yourself back onto the mat. Repeat 10 times, alternating legs.

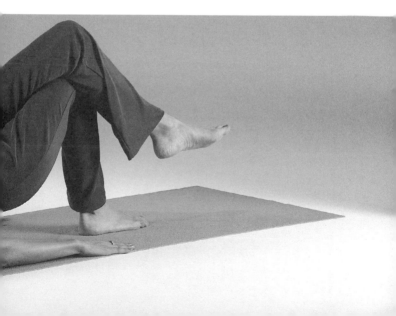

This is almost exactly like the cat stretch on page 98 – the only difference is that one hand is on your back reaching towards the diagonal shoulder blade.

Kneeling, make a square of the body. Keep your left hand under your left shoulder, fingers facing forwards. Place your other hand on your back and try to reach your diagonal shoulder blade. Knees should be hip-width apart. If your knees feel a little bit uncomfortable, just fold up a towel and put it under them. Place your feet gently on the floor and don't lock your elbow at any point during the stretch. As you breathe out, drop your chin to your chest and curl your stomach into your spine. Press your upper back to the ceiling, trying not to rock back and forth. As you breathe in, your tailbone lifts towards the ceiling, chest presses to the floor, and your head gently lifts. Breathe in, and reverse the position. Release into the "relaxation position" *(see page 110)* and just breathe. (Repeat four times on each arm.)

Watchpoints

■ Don't lock your elbows.

■ Don't lift your head too high or you may strain your neck.

■ As you press your chest down to the floor in the reverse exercise, if you feel any pinching in your lower back you've gone too far.

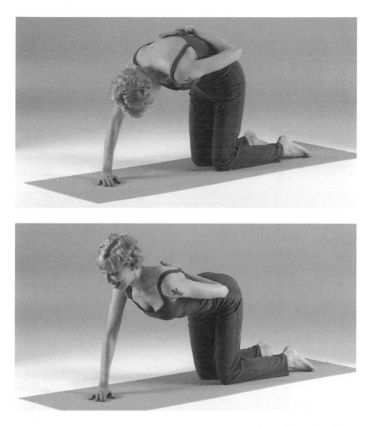

This exercise, and the two that follow, can either be done on the floor or sitting on a chair. This exercise works the shoulder joints and blades.

Sit comfortably. Breathe in, and slowly squeeze your right shoulder up to your right ear. Relax it down. Repeat with the other shoulder. Do this to a count of four up, four down. Don't move your head. Repeat 10 times, alternating shoulders.

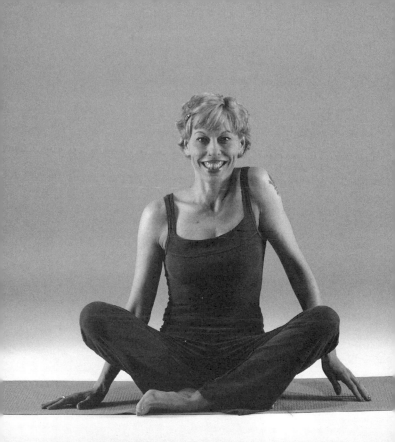

Sit comfortably on the floor or on a chair and squeeze both shoulders up to your ears. Make sure your hands are dangling loosely by your sides. If you feel you are arching your back, use a wall as support. Repeat 10 times.

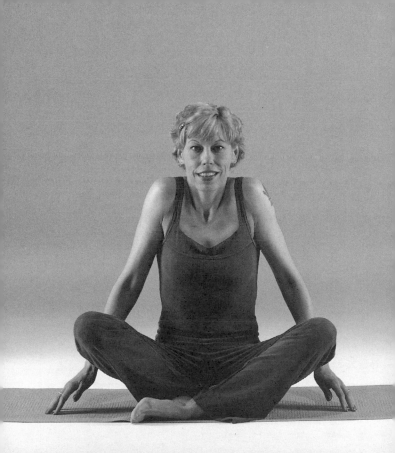

Assume the same position as the previous exercise. With
both your hands on your shoulders, very gently circle both
arms forward. Repeat 10 times. Then circle your arms
backwards and again, repeat 10 times. If this feels
uncomfortable, circle your shoulders with your arms at
your sides.

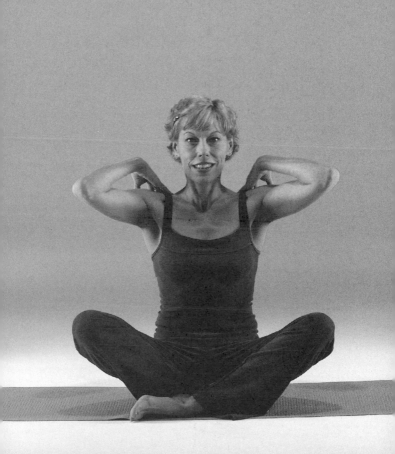

Lie on your stomach and imagine you're a small starfish.
Your arms are slightly wider than your shoulders, your
forehead on the floor on a folded towel. Make sure your
legs are comfortably apart and rotated slightly outwards.
Place your right arm on your back reaching towards the left
shoulder blade. Breathe out and let your left arm gently
float off the ground. As your arm reaches away, think of
your shoulder blade "gliding." You should feel this with the
hand on your back. Make sure that as your stomach goes
in, your pelvis drops. As you breathe out, don't grip your
bottom.

Repeat four times, first on one side then the other. Then go
into the relaxation position *(see page 110)*.

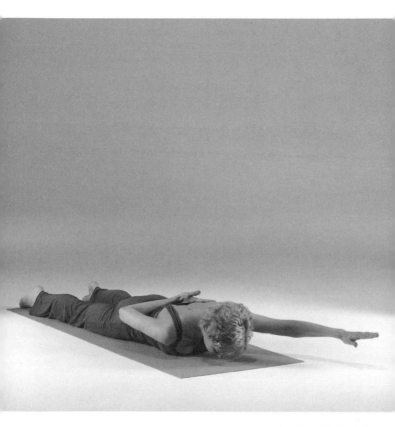

arm stretch against the wall

This exercise is done against a wall. This helps to stretch out the shoulder blades and the upper back.

Stand sideways on to a wall, about a foot away from it. Place your hand palm down on the wall. Do not arch your back. Very gently slide up the wall, leaning your body weight in to your palm, stretching your shoulder. Don't let the hips shift. Hold for a few seconds. Repeat four to six times, changing sides each time.

arm stretch against the wall 2

Stand facing the wall, with one hand on top of the other against it. Keep your stomach in, tailbone dropped. Don't stick your bottom out. Gently stretch up the wall. Hold for a few seconds. Repeat 10 times, changing the hand on top.

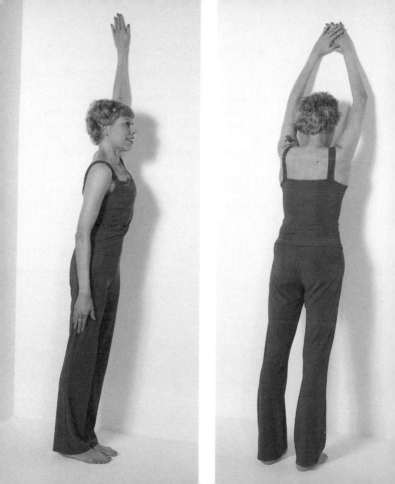

This exercise works the shoulders and shoulder blades.

Sit down on your heels in the relaxation position *(see page 110).* (If you find it difficult to kneel, you can sit on a chair and use a table to do it.) Have both hands wider than the shoulders and keep your head relaxed. Take a tennis ball in one hand and slowly, without moving anything else, lift that hand off the floor. Hold for a few seconds and relax back down. Don't twist your body or lift your head. You should feel your shoulder doing all the work. Change hands and repeat up to 10 times.

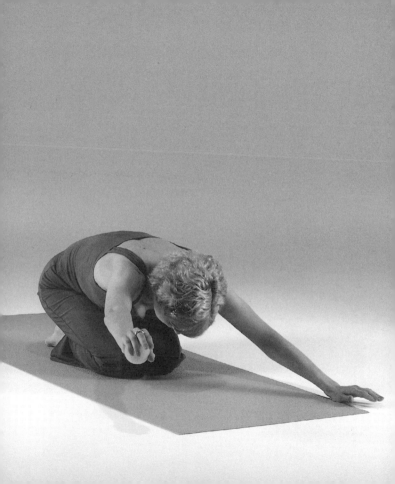

Assume the same position as in the previous exercise. This
time, keep the hand that you are not lifting behind your
back. Lift and relax as in the previous exercise. Change
hands and repeat up to 10 times.

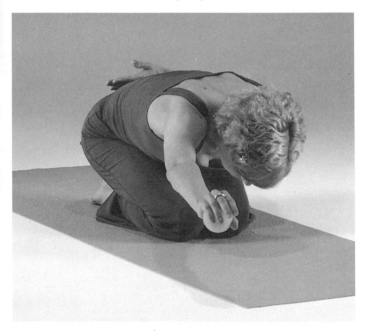

PART THREE

pilates with a ball

Physio Balls are an important tool in my Body Maintenance studio at Pineapple in London's Covent Garden. Currently available in sports stores, Physio Balls are a very simple exercise accessory that can be used almost anywhere – at the studio or at home, even in the office. They don't require a lot of space or time to blow them up; they're not a complicated piece of equipment.

the physio ball program

WHY USE A PHYSIO BALL?

Physio Balls have been a part of Body Maintenance for the last 10 years. When I first introduced them, they weren't widely known. Initially, I started using them in my Pilates-based technique because I had learned of their use in advanced physiotherapy taking place in German clinics.

A serious remedial tool, Physio Balls are especially important for patients recovering from surgery, particularly those recovering from spinal surgery. They have also been used at the New York City Ballet and, since then, have been successfully incorporated into most gyms and exercise regimes, where they have proved to be extremely useful.

In the Body Maintenance studio I have devised simple exercises for people recovering from spinal surgery. They are also fantastic for shoulder and spine problems, particularly scoliosis in the upper back. Amazingly, most of my clients now do at least 25 to 30 percent of their 90-minute program with a Physio Ball.

From the point of view of strengthening, stabilizing, and mobilizing your joints and muscles, Physio Balls are essential. However, it is worth remembering that for people with a serious problem or injury, the use of a Physio Ball must be undertaken only under the guidance of a qualified physiotherapist.

The exercises in this section are *not* remedial exercises. They are ordinary exercises that have been designed to offer you a varied and challenging program. The standing and balancing exercises can be used with or without a Physio Ball (a number of these can be found in the core exercise program on pages 67–173) although one of the many pluses of working on a ball is that the exercises are not done standing, so the correct posture can be more easily achieved.

The exercise routine featuring the ball is rigorous, but it does not place undue weight or pressure on the joints. These exercises allow you to focus more on correct posture and correct alignment, without having to worry about gravity in the way that you do when you are standing.

CORE STABILITY

One reason why Physio Balls are an essential tool in Body
Maintenance is that exercising with them increases *core
stability*. This is the utilization of the abdominals and the
muscles in the spine to create postural integrity that will
give you the posture and balance of someone who is much
younger and more confident. Better posture and balance
helps you to exude vitality and youthfulness.

On the unstable surface of a Physio Ball, the body works
harder to achieve the internal stability you would normally
get from doing basic abdominal exercises. When my older,
more mature clients work on a ball, they unconsciously
employ the many muscle groups that we normally don't use
to support the body.

Physio Balls also strengthen your "proprioceptive
awareness" – a popular concept in dance and bodywork.
This is the unconscious link between mind and body, the
physiological connection between the brain and the body.
For example, if your proprioceptive awareness is developed
and you slip on the street, you're more likely to regain your
balance than to lose it. Tripping or falling happen because
the lack of coordination between your mind and body has
increased your chances of losing your balance. The Body
Maintenance system of controlled, focused exercise works
on strengthening your proprioceptive awareness. Without
thought or analysis, the body corrects itself to avoid any
mishap or misstep.

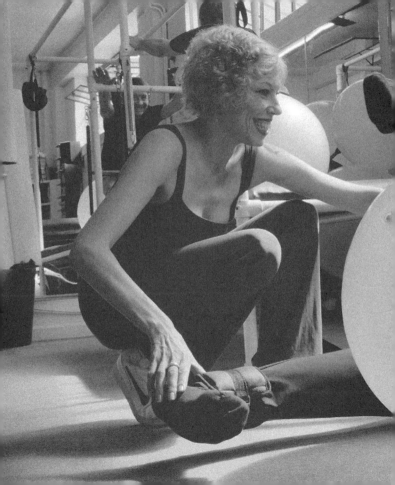

WHICH BALL?

Physio Balls come in different sizes. On the correct-sized ball for your height you should be able to sit with your hips and knees at a 90-degree angle. Anyone below 5ft 8in (173cm) tall should use a 55cm ball. Anyone 5ft 8in to 5 ft 9in (173cm to 176cm) should use a 65cm ball. Having said this, I would recommend that most people, except men over 6ft (182cm), should get a 55cm ball, because for most of the exercises, like press ups over the ball, you will want the smaller-sized ball.

Pump up the ball so that it feels firm and solid. If it feels soggy, you need to keep pumping, which is best done at a garage forecourt air-pump or by using a foot pump at home.

Precautions

The ball should not be placed anywhere near sharp objects or near heat. Do not allow children to play with it. Do not exercise wearing sharp objects like buckles or belts. Foremost, you need to remember that the ball is an unstable surface, so at the beginning of every exercise it is important to start near something or someplace you can actually hold on to. This is particularly important if you are pregnant or if you have any problems with instability in your spine or hips, or if you feel you have reached a certain age where you do not have good balance.

PREPARATION

Before you begin exercising with the ball, try this simple preliminary body awareness exercise.

Standing or sitting, close your eyes. Take a few deep breaths, then, starting with your head, slowly direct your focus down through your whole body. Visualize each part of your body as you imagine steering the flow of energy through it from part to part.

Visualize your eyes, ears, mouth, down your shoulders, arms, and hands.

Visualize your chest, back, abdomen, hips, pelvic area, upper legs, knees, lower legs, ankles, and feet.

As you visit each area, try to build up a mental picture of how it looks and feels. Spend a few seconds on each part. Move your head gently, shrug your shoulders. Gently move your stomach, tailbone, and hips. Concentrate on the sensation as you do this. Which areas feel most comfortable and relaxed? Are certain areas tight and constricted?

Now repeat, seated on the ball in the perfect posture position *(see page 272)*. Make sure to hold on to something if your eyes are closed.

Do this for a few minutes each day. It will help you to become more aware of your body when you are ready to begin the exercises.

Sequence of exercises

This is just a quick reminder of the guidance given in the main introduction. Start your exercise routine with the seated ball exercises before moving on to the floor exercises, because this way you will be working from a strong center. As well as doing some basic abdominal work, you should follow strengthening exercises with the relevant stretches. You can then alternate upper and lower body work each day.

The sequence:

1 Start with the balance and shoulder releases.
2 Move on to the pelvic tilt and abdominal exercises.
3 Follow with the back exercises.
4 Do leg exercises and stretches.
5 Finish with upper body exercises and stretches.

Now before you begin, flick back to page 64 and remind yourself of the safety instructions.

Correct breathing is an essential facet of Pilates. As you
breathe properly you will find it becomes much easier to
exercise. The problem is that most people don't breathe
deeply enough. Breathing slowly and deeply is very
energizing, as it ensures there is sufficient oxygen
circulating throughout the body.

It may sound obvious, but be careful not to hold your breath
when you exercise. It's better to breathe incorrectly than
not at all.

Practice this exercise before you start any stomach work.

basic breathing exercise

Seated on the ball, knees hip-width apart, arms hanging
loosely beside and slightly in front of your body, feel
relaxed, head "floating" upwards, relaxed on your neck.

- Place one hand on your stomach and very gently breathe in
  through your nose. Feel your lungs fill with oxygen and slowly
  expand and relax your stomach.
- With one finger on your pubic bone and one on your navel, try
  to shorten the gap between these two fingers as you breathe
  out, and flatten your stomach to your spine without moving
  the ball.
- Breathe in again and feel that gap slightly expand.

- Breathe out. Imagine there is a piece of string or an elastic band that links your pubic bone to your navel. Feel it very gently pulling up and in. This will make all three sets of stomach muscles work, including your oblique muscles, which will tighten your waist.

Try always to breathe slowly and deeply. One of the main rules of Pilates is to breathe out on the point of effort. If in doubt, particularly on the stretches – breathe naturally.

When you breathe in, your stomach gently expands. It should not, however, swell in an exaggerated way. Try to think of your ribcage expanding gently to the sides so that you're not just breathing into your throat and upper chest.

You may feel dizzy when you first start to breathe properly at the start of this exercise program. This is because you are taking in more oxygen than normal, as you are breathing more deeply, which can make you feel light-headed.

first movements

Seated on the ball, your tailbone heavy and both feet evenly placed on the floor, hip-width apart, try to be in contact from your center directly down through your feet into the floor. You are going to channel your energies from this center out through the crown of your head. Your shoulders and arms are relaxed. Your tailbone will drop and your abdominals will naturally pull back towards your spine. Try to think of your head sitting naturally on top of your shoulders, neither pushing it forward nor pulling it back.

Watchpoint

- If you force your shoulders back, and your lower back arches away from the ball, you know your shoulders are still too rounded for you to maintain this position and be anatomically correct.

Sitting in the same position as the previous exercise, squeeze both shoulders up to your ears. Make sure your hands are dangling loosely by your sides.

Repeat 10 times.

Watchpoint

- It is important not to lock your elbows or stick your chin forward.

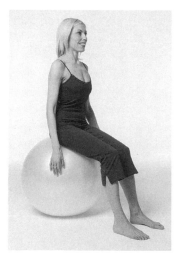
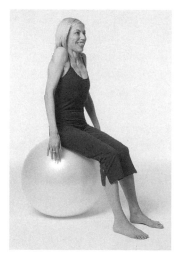

This exercise relaxes the shoulders and neck.

Sit comfortably on the ball with your arms relaxed at your sides. Breathe in, and slowly squeeze your right shoulder up to your right ear. Relax it down. Repeat with the other shoulder. Do this to a count of four up, four down. Don't move your head.

Repeat 10 times, alternating shoulders.

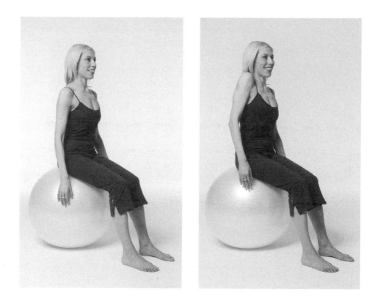

Assume the same position as in the previous exercise.
Place your hands on your shoulders and, very gently, circle
both arms forward.

Repeat 10 times.

Circle your arms backwards – again, repeat 10 times.

If this feels uncomfortable, you may have tight wrists: try
circling your shoulders with your arms hanging at your
sides.

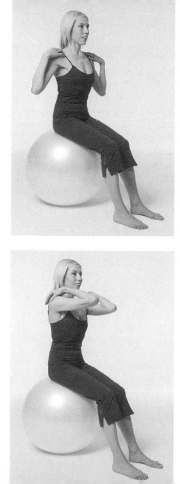

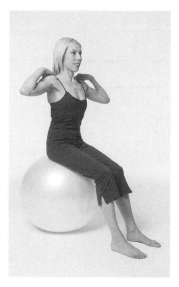

Seated on the ball, you can either have your fingers on your abdomen or allow your arms to hang naturally beside you. As you breathe in, your abdomen gently softens or expands into your fingers. As you breathe out, very gently let one foot float off the floor, feeling the connection of your navel to your spine. Place the foot down and ensure you have even pressure through both feet again. Then lift the other leg. Coordination is very important here. Start off Foot Lifts very slowly; eventually you will be able to do them faster so the interchange emanates from a stable pelvis and a strong abdomen.

Initially the change from one leg to the other might feel unstable, as you don't have the core strength to coordinate alternate leg lifts automatically. The feet should float off the floor.

Repeat for 10 lifts on each leg, alternating each time.

Watchpoints

- If you lift your feet too high, you will lose balance and wobble on the ball, as well as lose that postural alignment. Your tailbone will tuck underneath and your back will curl.

- Start with the ball close to something you can hold on to, like a chair, if you are worried about your balance.

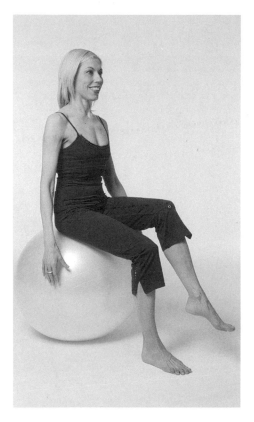

abdominal exercises

pelvic tilt

The pelvic tilt is a preparation exercise that warms up the back. It's a good starting point, whatever part of the program you plan to do.

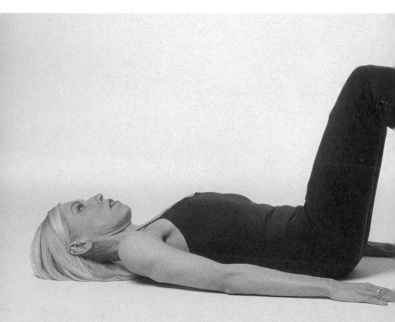

If you have high blood pressure, do not hold your breath in any of the bent-knee exercises. Keep your feet on the ball, knees and ankles in line, no pinching in the front of the hip and don't be too close to the ball.

Lie on your back with your knees bent and parallel, about hip-width apart with your feet on the ball supported against

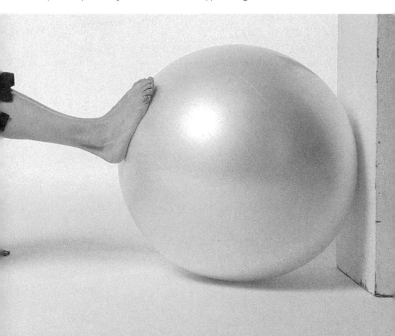

a wall. Your arms should be resting at your sides, with relaxed shoulders and palms facing the floor. This helps to lengthen your neck.

Breathe in, then breathe out and gently relax your back into the floor, your tailbone weighted on the mat. When you do this, do not press your back too strongly into the ground so that you lose your natural curve. Do not allow your back to arch to the point that it lifts off the floor. You want to maintain a neutral spine position, which is slightly different for each person. There is no point in trying to force your back down. Try very hard not to tense your buttock muscles during this exercise.

As you breathe out, gently tilt your pelvis forward and roll your lower back off the floor – one vertebra at a time, as you "peel" your back off the mat – until you are just below your shoulder blades. If you feel your ribs sticking forward or your neck shortening, you'll know you've gone too far.

Breathe in, keeping your neck long, and very slowly roll all the way down, breathing out, until your tailbone reaches the floor. Keep your feet relaxed on the ball and imagine your toes "lengthening" away.

Do approximately 10 repetitions.

Watchpoints

■ Keep your legs parallel to each other, and grip your bottom as little as possible.

■ There is a good chance you will feel this stretch in your calf and hamstrings. Don't worry about this unless it is really uncomfortable. If this is the case, skip this exercise.

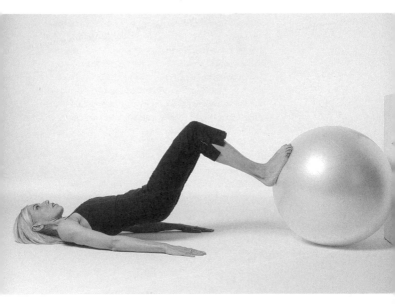

This is a preparation for the abdominal exercises. It will wake up your stomach muscles and prepare you for the more difficult exercises.

Secure the ball against a solid surface. Lie on the floor with your feet on the ball, with a relaxed back and long neck, without tucking your pelvis under. Take either a small cushion or folded towel and place it between your thighs.

Very gently breathe in through your nose. As you breathe out, feel your stomach muscles pulling down to the floor. Think of them pulling up and into your spine. Hold your breath and count to four. Squeeze the towel or cushion with your thighs, contracting your deep internal muscles. You can put your fingers on your stomach if you wish so that you can feel the muscles you are working.

As you breathe in through your nose, feel your stomach gently expand into your fingers. As you breathe out, feel your stomach pull away from your fingers. Feel your lower abdominal muscles working. Think of working on the transverse and the rectus abdominus muscles first, and the obliques second.

Repeat 10 times.

Watchpoints

- Don't let your pelvis lift off the floor. This will "shorten" your neck. Watch that your stomach doesn't "bloat." Instead, make sure that on the point of relaxation – when you breathe in – your stomach gently expands. As you breathe out you should feel your stomach pull up and in, away from the pubic bone.

- Most people naturally want to breathe in and pull their stomach muscles in – this is a mistake. As you breathe in, you gently soften the muscles as they flow out into your fingers. As you breathe out, the stomach pulls away from your fingers. Think of it as pulling "up and in." This will help you focus on your lower abdominals – strengthening and toning that area.

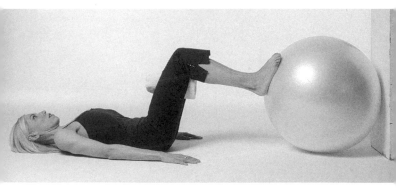

Lie in the same position as in the previous exercise, knees bent, legs together. You can place your hands on your hipbones. This helps to stabilize your pelvis.

Very gently breathe in and let your knees open to shoulder-width apart, making a small "V" shape. As you breathe out, feel the resistance. Bring your legs back together, focusing through your inner thighs as a passive resistance, breathing out and pulling your stomach in.

Repeat 10 times.

Watchpoints

- Think of the muscles between your navel and your pubic bone as a fan. As you inhale and your knees open to the side, the fan opens. As you exhale, the muscles tighten and the fan closes.

- Don't press your back into the floor.

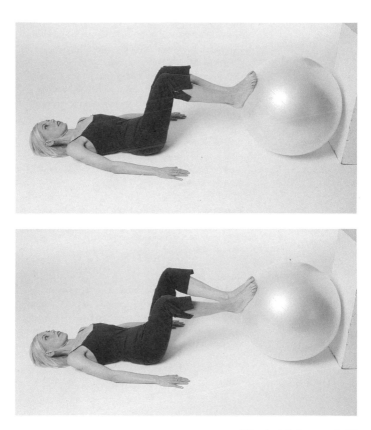

This slightly harder version of the previous exercise is very straightforward. Interlace your hands behind your head (this will help prevent you from straining the muscles in your neck). Slide them high up behind your skull. Do not let them slip to your neck. Keep your thumbs on either side of your spine. Don't stick your chin out.

Lift your elbows so that you can just see them out of the corner of your eye without moving your head. When you can see your elbows peripherally you know that your arms are in the right place.

Very gently exhale and "float" your head and shoulders off the mat. As you lift, squeeze your legs together, inhale and lower your head and shoulders, opening your legs again. Repeat 10 times.

Watchpoint

- As you lift your head your focus shouldn't change, so you don't shorten your neck. If you shorten your neck, you may tip your pelvis. This makes it very hard to work your lower abdominal muscles. You may also place a strain on your lower back and your body will be incorrectly aligned.

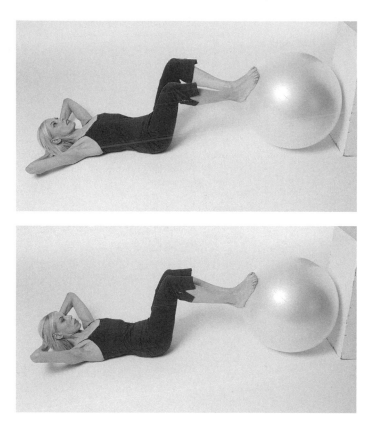

This exercise uses exactly the same position as the previous exercise, although your feet and knees should be hip-width apart. All the same rules apply. Keeping your feet on the ball, lift your elbows up to where you can see them in your peripheral vision. Keep looking at the ceiling and gently breathe in through your nose. Relax your abdomen, but do not "bloat" it out.

As you breathe out, gently lift your head and shoulders off the mat. Only go as high as you can. Do not strain your neck to hold the position.

Breathe in as you go back down again.

Watchpoint

■ As you breathe out, imagine that a piece of string is pulling you up from the pubic bone and under your ribcage. Pause until all three sets of abdominal muscles go "up and in," and flatten.

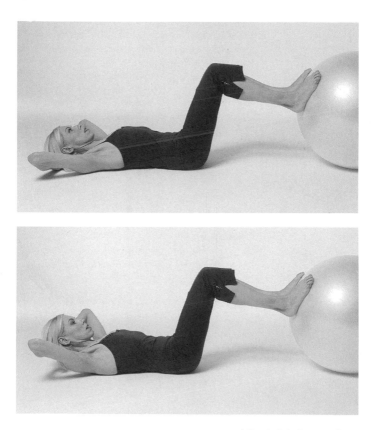

Lie on your back with your hands on your hips or on the
floor and your calves on the ball, keeping your legs
comfortably externally rotated in the hip socket.

As you breathe out, lift your left leg, pulling up through the
inside thigh, and pulling in through the lower abdominals.

Breathe in as you lower your leg.

Breathe out and lift your right leg.

Do not lift too high. Only lift as high as you feel comfortable
with in the hamstrings in the back of your leg.

Watchpoint

- If you keep your hands on your hips this will ensure you don't
  lift too high, as you will otherwise pinch into your hip.

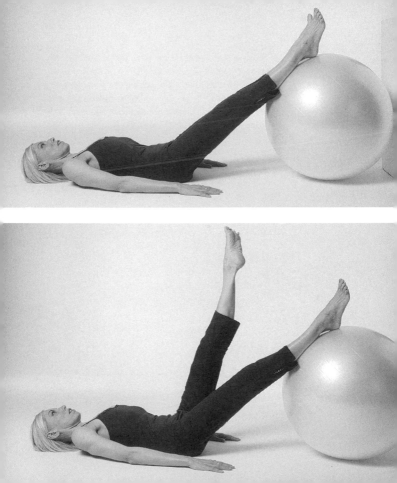

To make this exercise harder, do exactly the same routine but add a small sit-up into the lift, making it a more coordinated exercise. So, as you breathe out and lift your leg, curl forward in a similar way to the earlier abdominal curl exercise, and breathe in as you lower both your leg and upper body.

Do a maximum of 10 repetitions of both exercises, five on each leg, alternating each time.

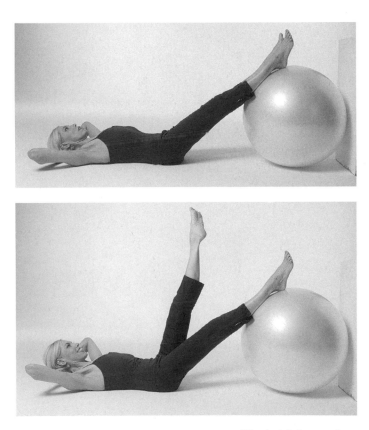

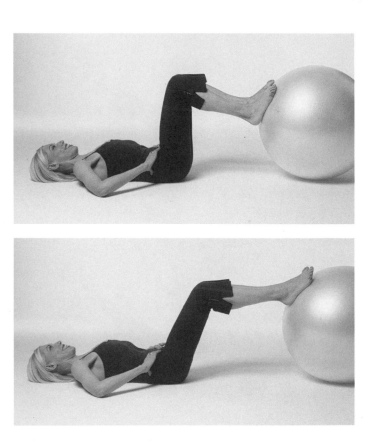

Lie in the starting position as for the abdominal preparation
exercises *(see page 284).* The ball is unsupported in this
exercise. The feet are comfortably positioned on the ball,
with your hips and knees in line, and hands on your hips.
Everybody tends to reverse this excrcise, so it is very
important to concentrate. It is a small movement.

As you breathe in, push the ball away from you – about half
a meter or a foot.

As you breathe out, draw the ball towards you using your
lower abdominals, particularly the transverse abdominus,
which are between your hipbones (the ones you use in the
fanning exercise).

Two common mistakes can happen: If you push the ball too
far away, your back will arch and you will feel uncomfortable
as you breathe in. If as you breathe out you draw the ball in
too far, you will pinch your hips. Your hands will tell you if
you've come too far.

Repeat 10 times.

This exercise and the one following it are the most advanced in the abdominal sequence. If you have any lower back problems at all, I suggest that you leave these two exercises until you feel strong enough.

Lie on your back with the ball between your calves, keeping your knees relaxed. You want the ball to be reasonably close to you. If you feel your lower back arching, bring the ball closer. However, you don't want the ball so close that your bottom leaves the floor. It is difficult to recommend exactly the position of your legs, because this varies from person to person. You want to feel secure, with your lower back supported.

Leaving the ball suspended in the air between your calves, the exercise is similar to the basic abdominal curl.

Breathe out and curl forward, engaging your navel to your spine. Breathe in as you lower yourself.

If you find this exercise is very demanding you can start with four repetitions and slowly build up to 10.

Watchpoints
■ When lifting your legs, bend your knees as you place the ball between your calves. When you lower your legs, take the ball from your calves with your hands and then bend your knees as you put your feet back on the ground.

■ Never lift from or lower the ball to the ground using your legs. Take the ball in your hands and "position" the ball on the way up, and remove the ball before returning your feet to the ground.

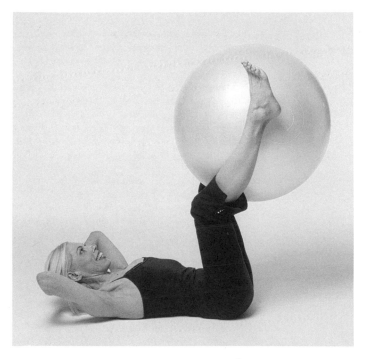

The last exercise for the abdominals is again a challenging one, working the obliques, which are the muscles that support your waist. It is a great waist-toning exercise.

Lying on your side in a straight line, position the ball between your calves. Bring your legs slightly forwards and ensure you do not have an arch in your lower back. Breathe in.

As you breathe out, lift your legs off the ground, pulling your stomach in. As you lift your legs, you want to draw the "underneath" part of your waist off the mat. If your underneath waist and hip are sinking into the mat, you have lifted too far. If you have any discomfort in your lower back at all, bring your legs further forwards.

Do 10 repetitions, alternating sides.

If you have any worries about your back at all, build up to this exercise (and the previous one) over a period of weeks or months.

Watchpoint

- If this is the first time you are doing this exercise, even possibly the first four times, I suggest that you lie on your side with your back against a wall so you can feel your middle back supported by the wall. Having your middle back supported will give you a clearer proprioceptive sense of spinal integrity.

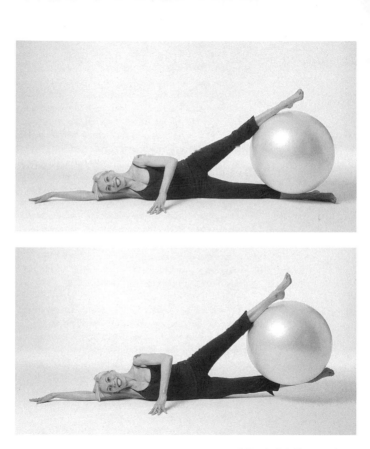

cat stretch

This exercise will release your lower back and stretch out your shoulders. The cat stretch is essential for spinal health, as it works equally on flexion and extension, both essential functions for a healthy spine.

If you wish, support the ball against the wall. Kneel as far away as you can while still resting your palms on the ball. Your weight should be distributed evenly through both knees. Your hips should be in line with your knees. Breathe out, curl your chin into your chest, stomach into your spine, and stretch out your lower back, from the inside out, drawing all your internal organs into your spine. You get the blood flowing as you open your spine, and this will counteract the effects of being seated for long periods of time.

As you breathe in, press your chest down, your bottom up, and gently lengthen your neck and head, stretching out tight shoulders and the upper thoracic spine. This counts as one repetition. Repeat 10 times.

Watchpoints
- If you feel your neck crunching or your vocal chords contracting you've taken your head too far back. There should be no discomfort in your neck.
- Make sure your feet stay on the floor.

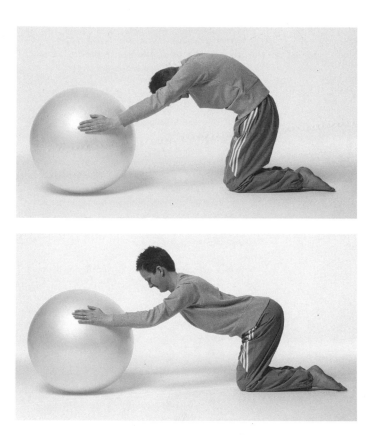

This exercise helps improve balance, stabilizes the pelvis, and strengthens the spine and abdominal muscles.

Rest the ball under your stomach with your feet on the floor, legs straight and hands in front of you shoulder-width apart. The spine is neutral and the stomach gently in.

Breathe in and, as you breathe out, let your right arm and left leg gently float away. Don't lift too high or your hip will leave the ball. To avoid this, position something like a kitchen roll across the base of your spine. If you lift too high, it will fall off. Keep your pelvis neutral, so that you don't tilt from side to side. Keep looking at the same point on the floor, so that you don't shorten your neck. Relax back into the starting position.

Repeat, alternating arms and legs, for 10 repetitions.

Watchpoint
■ If this exercise feels too difficult at the onset, you can start by lifting one arm or one leg only, rather than both together at the same time.

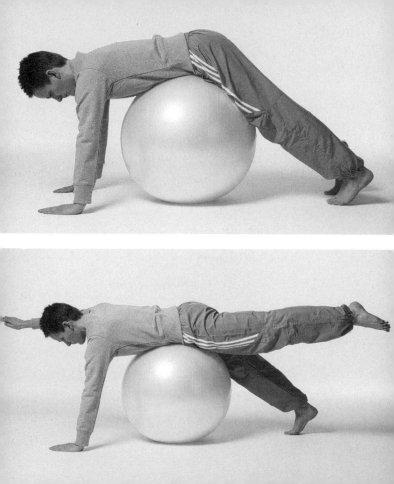

You may feel more stable wearing trainers for this exercise. Have your feet based against a secure surface like a wall. Position your legs hip-width apart, securely against the wall. Relax over the ball with your hips against the ball and your hands behind your back. Breathe in.

As you breathe out, curl forward on flexion, pulling your stomach in. Extend to a straight back, pause, then breathe in.

Breathe out and reverse the curl. This is similar to a cat stretch.

Watchpoints

- As you curl forward, keep looking at the same point unless you have a very flexible spine.

- You may feel your hamstrings tightening a certain amount, but you don't want to stabilize yourself by gripping your buttock. Keep the buttock muscles relaxed.

- Ensure that your shoulders are also relaxed, and do not lift them up to your ears. Keep your head and neck in line. If you lift your head too far and take it behind you, you will shorten the muscles in your neck. You will know if you are doing the exercise incorrectly if you feel pinching in your lower back or in your neck.

- If you go too far and your stomach bulges out, you will not be strengthening your back but weakening it.

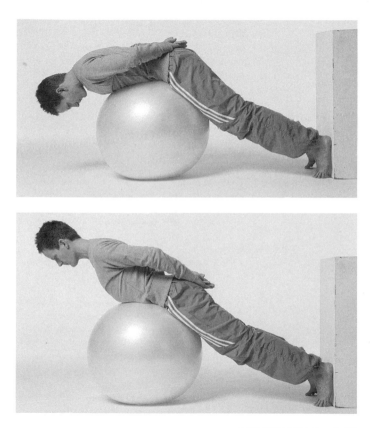

In my studio I call this the Flying Swan. Obviously it is a very demanding exercise for the abdominals and the spine, therefore you have to be secure in your balance.

Start in the same position as the previous back exercise, but move away from the wall. Position the ball under your hips and breathe in.

As you breathe out, tip the ball forward so you are resting on the palms of your hands, your legs in the air behind you. Breathe in. Breathe out, reverse the movement, and let your feet come on to the floor and your arms float above your head, shoulder-width apart. This movement counts as one repetition. Start with four and build up to a maximum of 10.

Watchpoints

- Many people wear trainers for this exercise to stabilize their legs so they don't slip.

- As with all back exercises, the stomach is the instigator of the movement. As you breathe out your stomach goes in, the shoulders are relaxed, and the buttocks are not tensed.

- Make sure that as your stomach goes in, your pelvis relaxes back. As you breathe in, don't grip your bottom.

- Keep your legs straight. If you bend your knees, the exercise won't be as effective.

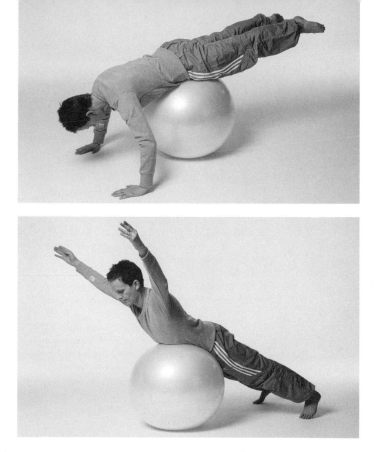

Lie on your back with your feet on the ball, feet and legs together and your tailbone on the floor. Your ankles and knees should be in line with your hips, your feet relaxed. Breathe in.

As you breathe out, move your legs one way, your head the other way – your stomach should remain stable.

Breathe in and come back to the center.

Repeat in the opposite direction.

Watchpoints

- The most important part of this exercise is that at no point should either shoulder blade leave the mat.

- Your knees should stay together as you move from side to side – this way one leg won't get longer than the other.

- It is very natural as you move from side to side to take the knees further than the ankles – the movement is taken from the abdominals as the legs and the ball go from side to side. This is a small movement. Do not let the ball take you further over than your abdominals can control the movement.

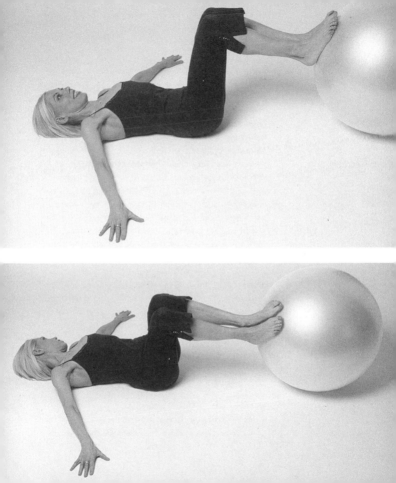

toning and stretching your legs

inside thigh Lift

This exercise will help tone your inner thighs. You do it lying on your side, either with your hand supporting your head or with your arm completely flat. If you choose to keep your arm flat, it may feel more comfortable to put a towel between your arm and ear. The other hand is in front of you. Your top leg should be forward, in front of your body, with your foot on the ball. The underneath leg (the one that is working) needs to be slightly forward, with your foot gently flexed. Don't lock the knee, but pull up the muscles so that your leg is straight. If your legs are not straight, you'll be working your ankle and your foot much more than your inner thigh.

Breathe in and then, as you breathe out, lift your "underneath" leg and hold. Then slowly lower it. Don't lift your leg too high. Think of your leg as going "away," not up – you want to lengthen and strengthen your muscles, not have them contracted and tight. As you lift and breathe out, your stomach pulls in, just like in the earlier stomach exercises. The energy is through the heel, working your inside thigh. Do 10 on each side.

Watchpoints

■ It's important to remember that, in all the leg exercises, the instigator is your stomach. This means you should feel your abdominal muscles working. The same applies to all the upper body exercises.

- Make sure your hips are stacked one on top of the other.
- You can use a wall to make sure your back is in the correct position. If in doubt, bring the underneath leg forward.

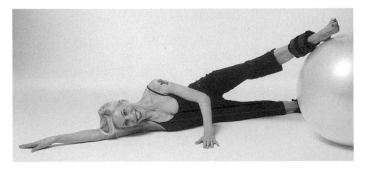

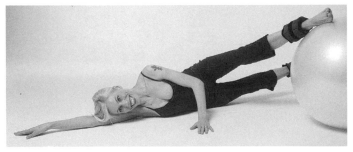

Lie on your side as in the previous exercise.

Breathe in and, as you breathe out, lift the underneath leg, bend the knee gently, and then squeeze to straighten it. The foot is gently flexed, the knee is not locked, and keep your abdominals in towards your spine.

Do 10 repetitions on each side, keeping your leg in the air the whole time.

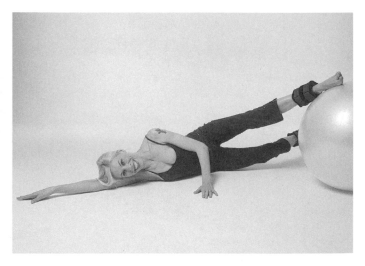

Lie on your front, position the ball comfortably between your
ribs and hips, arms shoulder-width apart, neck in line, legs
hip-width apart, feet on the floor and flexed for balance. Do
not lock your elbows, and keep your wrists in line.

Keeping your foot softly flexed so as to engage the correct
muscles, very gently breathe in, then breathe out and lift
your leg. Then slowly bring it down, keeping the buttocks
tightly gripped. Do 10 repetitions on each leg.

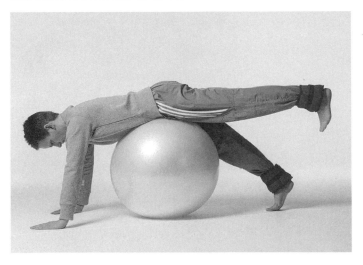

Assume the same position as in the previous exercise, still keeping your feet softly flexed. Breathe in, then very gently breathe out and lift both legs up. Slowly bring them down, remembering to keep the buttocks gripped. Do 10 repetitions.

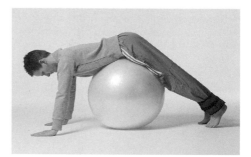

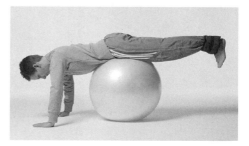

All the same rules apply as the exercise on page 315.
Starting in the same position, this time lift one leg off the
floor to parallel with your hip, flexing your foot as you lift.
Bend at the knee so your ankle and knee are in line.
Squeeze and lift the leg 10 times, keeping your hip on
the ball so as not to distort your pelvis. Repeat with the
other leg.

Watchpoints

- At no point in any of these bottom-toning exercises should
  your hipbones leave the ball.

- If you feel discomfort in your lower back, adjust your position
  slightly over the ball, alternatively do not lift your legs so high
  to begin with. Very occasionally people feel nauseous lying
  over a ball, so be aware of this.

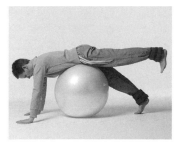 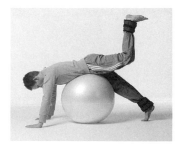

Lean forward over the ball with your hands firmly on the floor and your feet on the ground. Keep your shoulders relaxed. Breathe in and very gently "grip" (tighten) your bottom. As you do so, you should feel your stomach going in and your tailbone drop.

Exhaling, raise your right leg and flex your foot. Then gently inhale and bend your leg, keeping your buttocks squeezed at all times. Exhale and straighten the leg, keeping it in the air for 10 repetitions, breathing in as you bend it, and out as you straighten it. Repeat with the other leg.

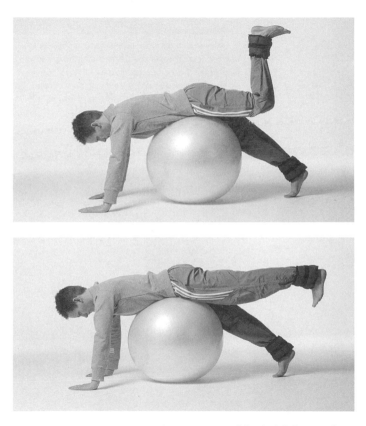

Stand up straight using the ball as a support against a
wall, hands comfortably apart. Take a step forward with
your left leg and, leaning against the ball, bend the knee
slightly and feel the stretch down through your right leg.
Keep your right heel down. Do not bounce. Hold for 30
seconds. Repeat four times, alternating legs.

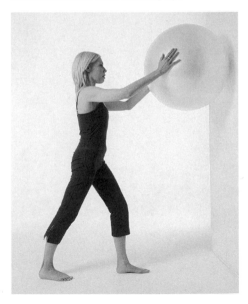

This exercise will help to release your hips.

Lying on your back with your legs bent and feet resting on the ball, supported by a wall, very gently cross your right ankle over the left knee. Make sure it's the ankle, and not the toes. Use your right hand to press your left knee towards the ball, making sure your hips do not twist. Remember, you should feel a stretch only in the working leg. Hold for 30 seconds, change legs and repeat four times.

Watchpoint

■ Make sure your tailbone stays on the floor.

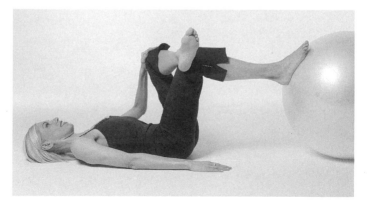

Kneel down on your right leg, keeping your back straight
and with your hands resting on the ball supported by a wall.
Extend your left leg, making sure that your heel is always in
front of your knee. Gently pull your stomach in and lean
back slightly, making sure you don't arch your back. Hold
for 30 seconds. Repeat twice for each leg.

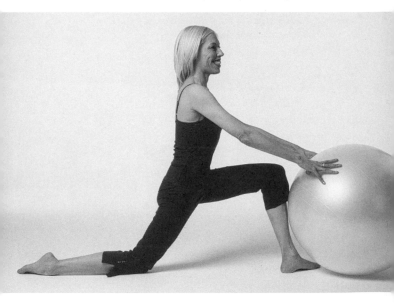

To make this exercise more challenging, take one hand off the ball and use it to take hold of your back ankle and draw it towards your bottom.

Watchpoint

■ If this stretch causes any pain in your knee or back, stop at once.

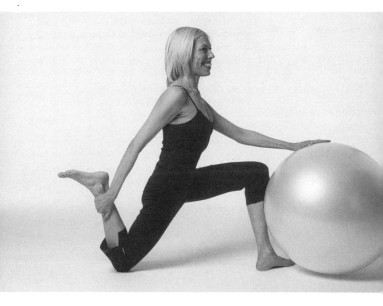

For this exercise, most people need to place a towel
beneath their head. Lie on your mat or towel.

Resting your feet on the ball supported by a wall, knees
bent, make sure you have equal weight down through both
feet. Your arms are beside you and your pelvis is in the
neutral position. Very gently bend your right knee into your
chest. Grasp the back of your thigh with your left hand.
Grasp the back of your calf with your right hand and gently
unfold, straightening that leg with a flexed foot, and ease
the leg towards you, moving your left hand up to your calf.

Do the right, then the left leg, and repeat, a minimum of
twice on each side, holding for 30 seconds each time.

Watchpoints

- You'll know you are doing this wrong if your bottom lifts. If
  you find it impossible to hold your leg with your hands, take a
  towel, place it around your calf and ease the leg towards you,
  keeping your neck and shoulders relaxed.

- Don't pull on your leg so that your bottom leaves the floor, as
  your pelvis will twist. You want to flex the foot without overly
  tensing the feet, and gently straighten that knee. It is more
  important to get your knee straighter than to bring the leg
  closer to you.

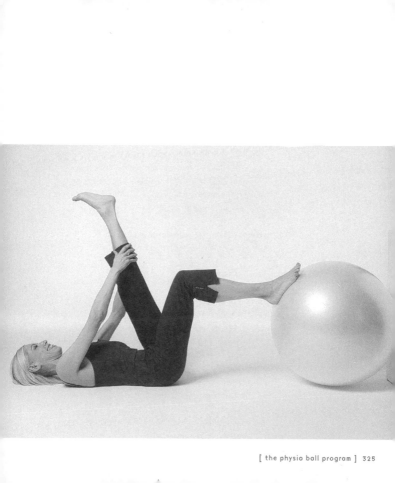

upper body toning

Now you're ready to continue with your upper body toning
and strengthening. Kneel down with your hands on the floor
in front of the ball, and feet behind the ball. Carefully walk
forwards until your hips are on the ball and feet off the
floor. Your hands are under your shoulders – just wider than
shoulder-width apart, with the palms flat and fingers
pointing away from you. Keeping your head in line, gently tip
your weight forwards.

Breathe in as you bend the arms, breathe out as you
straighten them, engaging your navel towards your spine.

Repeat 10 times.

Watchpoints

■ The alignment of your neck and upper back is essential. Try
not to seesaw and let your legs go up and down. As well as
toning arms and upper back, this is essential for core
stability and abdominal control.

■ The further over the ball you are, the less stable you are and
the harder you have to work to stop your back arching.

■ Keep your legs together and your inner thighs gently
squeezed to feel more stable.

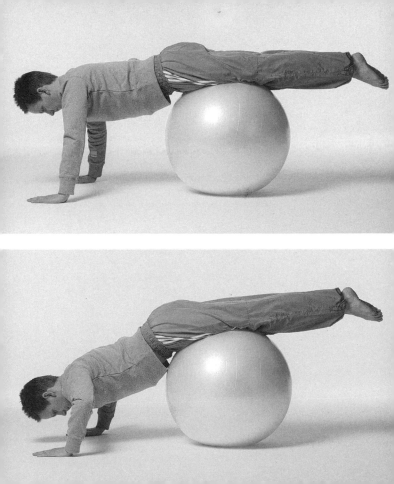

You will need a hand-weight for this one (if you haven't got one, a can of beans or plastic bottle of water will do).

Place your right hand on the ball and kneel behind it, your left arm holding the weight. Keep your neck in line with the rest of your body. Holding the hand-weight, breathe in as you lift your left elbow up as high as you can, keeping the elbow bent at a right angle, without twisting your body. Exhale as you straighten your arm behind you. Pause. Bend your arm back again. Repeat 10–15 times on each arm (one set). If you like you may do a second set.

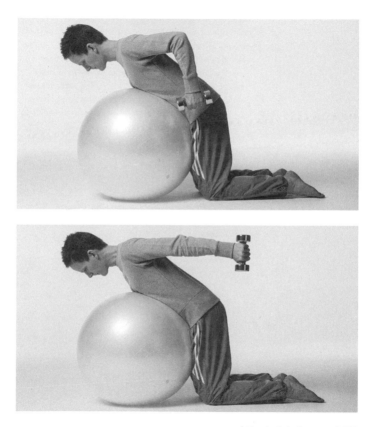

Sit on the ball with a two-kilo weight in each hand, breathe in and bend your right arm up to shoulder level. Breathe out and straighten to waist level. Try not to rock from side to side as you do this. Repeat 10 to 15 times with alternate arms. It is better to start with lighter weights if you have any doubts about the strength in your neck and shoulders.

To make this upper body sequence harder, slowly build to two sets of three exercises: 15 press-ups, 15 triceps presses on each arm, and 15 bicep curls on each arm.

Watchpoint

- At no point allow your back to arch – the focus is firstly abdominal stability and then toning the relevant muscle groups.

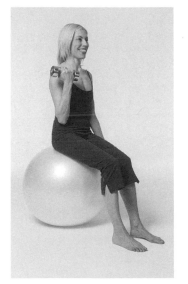

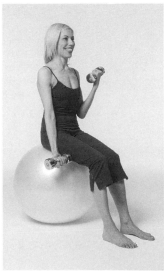

After upper body strengthening, it is important to stretch out your shoulders. Sit in correct alignment on the ball.

Holding your arms up in front of your face, cross one over the other and clasp your hands together. Then gently push your elbows to the ceiling and feel your shoulders stretching apart. As you raise your arms, keep your shoulders down and hold this position for a count of 10. Repeat this stretch four times, alternating arms.

We are now going to do shoulder stretches with the ball in a kneeling position. For those of you who have any discomfort in your knees or lower back, I have included an exercise (alternative double shoulder stretch, page 338) where you push the ball up a wall instead.

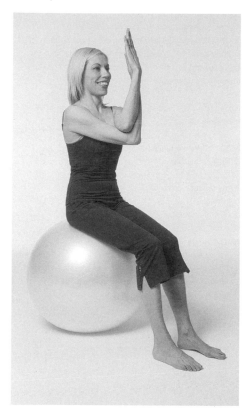

For this first shoulder stretch, you are kneeling down. Your bottom is resting on your heels. If you feel you have very tight feet and your feet are uncomfortable, you can put a towel under your feet.

Place the palm of your right hand on the center of the ball and breathe in.

As you breathe out, push the ball as far as it will go without lifting your bottom.

Breathe in and come back to an upright position.

Do 10 repetitions on each arm.

Watchpoints

■ As you breathe out, feel the shoulder stretching, the shoulder blade gliding up towards your ear, then relaxing back as you breathe in. Your head and neck should just flow along the arm in a relaxed, soft movement. If your neck feels uncomfortable, you are probably in the wrong position, so adjust until your neck feels comfortable.

■ Your elbow should not be locked at any point.

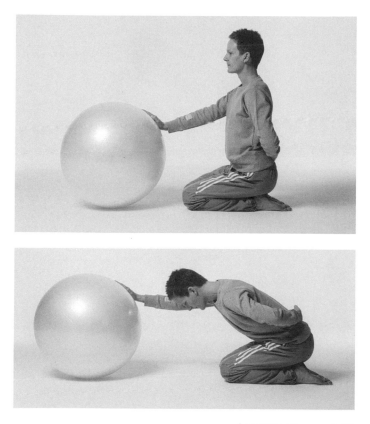

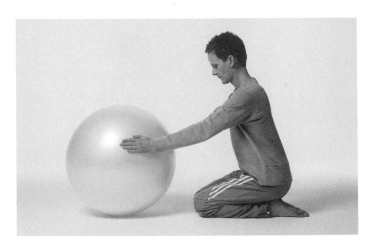

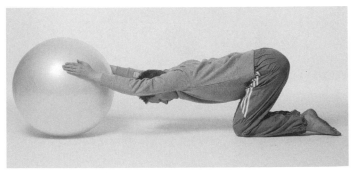

double shoulder stretch

The next exercise is much more challenging. Start in the
same position as the single shoulder stretch, but place
both hands on the ball. Breathe in then, as you breathe
out, push the ball away from you and your chest towards
the floor, lifting your bottom off your heels. Breathe in and
come back.

Repeat 10 times.

Watchpoints

■ Your ears should be relaxed between your arms the whole
   time. Most people drop their head too low. It's just as
   important not to lift your head too high, so that you feel a
   pinching in your neck.

■ If you feel any discomfort in your lower back, you are pushing
   the ball too far away.

■ Do not let your feet leave the ground.

This is the alternative to the previous kneeling exercise, and is useful for anyone with either bad knees or a serious lumbar condition. It is exactly the same exercise except that you are pushing the ball up a wall.

Stand with complete Pilates postural integrity, feet hip-width apart, stomach in, tailbone dropped, head and neck in line, arms raised with your ears between your arms, elbows released. Breathe in.

As you breathe out, push the ball up the wall. Make sure your abdominals are engaged so there is no arching in your lower back.

Repeat 10 times.

Watchpoint

- If you are too far away from the wall your heels will come off the ground and your back will arch. If you are too close you will not feel the stretch.

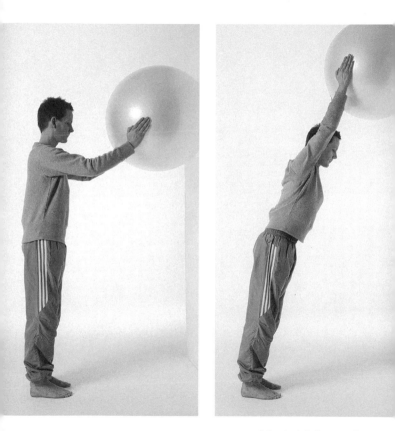

In the Body Maintenance studio, working with Physio Balls has been particularly useful for my pregnant clients. The Body Maintenance studio specializes in post- and antenatal work, and we teach pregnant clients right up until a week or two before birth; we also see them anywhere from six weeks after giving birth.

exercising during pregnancy

This section has been specifically devoted to the weekly exercise program performed by 10 to 15 of my clients in the Body Maintenance studio. You can be confident that they have been tried and tested successfully for a number of years by many women before and after they give birth, week in and week out – some even after their third or fourth child, or after having given birth to twins.

On an average week the studio can have anywhere between 10 and 15 clients who are expecting a baby. And after a certain period they all come back, usually between three and six months after the birth, to get their bodies back in shape.

The exercises shown in this book are only the sequence of exercises we do using the ball. In the studio we do a lot of other equipment-based work and mat work.

I cannot stress how important it is to realize that each pregnancy is different. Whether it is your first or your fourth or more, you must always listen to what your body is telling you. If you are tired at any point, rest. If you are hungry, eat. As I say to all my pregnant clients, the most important thing is a healthy mother and baby.

Exercises that may be perfectly fine one day may feel uncomfortable the next. This depends a lot on the way the baby is lying. Obviously, as the pregnancy develops you must listen to your body and if any exercise makes you feel uncomfortable you must stop. If you get any discomfort, particularly around the base of your abdominals, around your pubic bone, or your pelvic floor muscles, that is an indication that you need to stop exercising.

It is important only to exercise after first checking with your physician and any other healthcare professionals you may be seeing during your pregnancy. I feel it is necessary also to stress that if it is your first baby then you are much less aware of your body – any discomfort, nausea, any of the changes that the body naturally undergoes during pregnancy. In my studio – and physicians will also advise this – it is recommended that for up to the first three months you should not undertake a new exercise program. The risk of miscarriage is always higher during the first three months of pregnancy. Obviously, if your healthcare professional suggests that you do something, for instance swimming, that is a different issue. In my studio the clients who are pregnant always have priority of both my and my staff's attention. If you have any doubts at all about any of the exercises, I would much prefer you didn't do them.

Particularly for women in modern society, pregnancy realistically is a very small part of life. It is important not to pressurize yourself to keep fit, to overexercise, to worry about the shape of your body. Yes, you are having a baby. This means you are going to get larger. It is totally feasible to regain your body shape after pregnancy without worrying unduly about media images of pregnancy. Whenever any of my clients says, "I'm fat," I say, "You are not fat, you are pregnant." I will restate that a healthy mother and baby is what we all desire.

After the birth I always insist that my clients do not exercise until they have had their six-week check-up. This does not mean that you shouldn't do the pelvic floor exercises that your healthcare professionals give you (which they normally do) under their personal direction. What I am saying is that until you have had your six-week check-up your body is still at a vulnerable point and you need to take extra care of yourself. This also involves avoiding anything like heavy lifting, because your body is still under stress from the birth.

The relaxin hormones can still be in your body for up to a year after the birth of your baby, so it is important to tailor your exercise program with this in mind. You may feel fine now, but you may want to think about how your body may feel in 10 years if you overstress it when it is still vulnerable to the after-effects of childbirth. I cannot stress too strongly that the media images of women getting their bodies back in shape immediately after birth are *not* the norm. Some of my clients return to their natural shape within three months, some take six to eight months.

This depends on the individual concerned. Also, the older you are the harder it is for the body to bounce back.

It is also quite important to remember that it is very difficult to get back to what you might think of as your pre-pregnancy weight if you are breastfeeding. As we know, nursing is an essential part of a child's development. Most of my clients who breastfeed don't actually return to their natural weight until slightly after those who, for whatever reason, haven't breastfed their babies. If you are nursing, obviously you have to eat more because you are feeding yourself *and* the baby.

Every pregnancy is different, every birth is different, and every body is different, so it is important not to have unreal images of what you expect your body to look like before or after the birth. The main thing I want to stress is that you should be able to enjoy this phase of your life. You have made a positive choice to have a baby and it should be a joyous experience.

PILATES AND PREGNANCY
Jane Ireland MCSP SRP, Chartered Physiotherapist

For a mother, the birth of a child is a truly miraculous event. What I find even more remarkable are the physiological changes the body goes through from conception to birth, and how the mother's body recovers afterwards.

Pregnancy is not a disease or an illness, it is a condition which should be managed for the sake of the baby's development and the mother's wellbeing. A mother who is suffering from low back pain, pelvic instability, upper back or arm pain will not enjoy looking after her newborn baby.

Pregnancy puts great physical demands on the mother's body. Effective Pilates during and after pregnancy helps to support the body physically during pregnancy, and vitally helps the physical recovery afterwards.

From the early days of pregnancy, a hormone called *relaxin* is released into the body to help with the "softening" of the ligaments. This enables the mother's body to "grow" comfortably to accommodate the increasingly large fetus. With increasing laxity in the body ligaments, the joints are more vulnerable to the normal stresses and strains of everyday life. The mother's necessary increase in weight is also loading up her frame.

The human muscle system is trainable – that is, we can make it work to our advantage to help give stability and strength to a mother's body. However, it must be recognized that *not all exercise is beneficial.*

Pilates works on all muscle groups in a biomechanically correct way, so preventing overworking of some muscle groups and underworking of others, which can lead to an imbalanced muscle system and one which is prone to injury.

The basis of all Pilates is core stability (co-contracting of the pelvic floor and deep abdominal muscles). These muscles help control the pelvis and give support to the spine. Core stability exercises do not mean sit-ups; it is potentially dangerous to do sit-ups while pregnant. Lesley makes you work the core muscles in various challenging ways without putting you or your baby at risk.

Pregnancy often causes the mother's posture to change to more of a swaying-forward, slouched-shoulders presentation. This again makes you more vulnerable to pain and injury. Posture is constantly worked on at the Body Maintenance studio, both with strength work, flexibility, and body awareness.

Immediately after the birth of your child, gentle pelvic floor exercises should be started, but for any other exercise you should wait a minimum of six weeks. Pilates post-pregnancy will help to get your pelvic floor and abdominal control back; it will help to stabilize your spine, strengthen your upper body to help with the continual lifting of the baby, and – probably most noticeably of all – it will help you to get your body shape back!

I started doing Pilates at Body Maintenance just before my second pregnancy. I continued throughout the pregnancy, working on, among other things, core muscles, spinal strength and flexibility, leg strength and flexibility, arm strength and postural exercises. After my son was born I started again, initially with just a few exercises at home concentrating on the pelvic floor, then, as time allowed, in the studio. Lesley works you hard, and the work is extremely effective. Each individual program is designed to each woman's particular needs. The rewards are plenty: my body shape has come back – something I never thought would happen, having had two rather large baby boys! I feel stronger than I have in a long time, my posture is better, and I feel better in myself. Lesley – thank you.

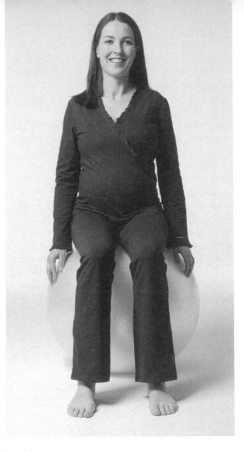

first movements

For this first exercise you are seated on the ball, your tailbone heavy and both feet evenly placed on the floor, hip-width apart. You are in contact from your center directly down through your feet into the floor. You are going to channel your energies from your center out through the crown of your head. Your shoulders and arms are relaxed. Your tailbone will relax and your abdominals will naturally drop back towards your spine.

Rather than pulling your tummy in, imagine the baby dropping back into your spine. Try to think of your head sitting naturally on top of your shoulders, neither pushing it forward nor pulling it back.

Gently bounce on the ball for anywhere up to three minutes.

These relax your shoulders and neck.

Sit comfortably on the ball with your arms relaxed at your sides. Breathe in and slowly squeeze your right shoulder up to your right ear. Breathe out and relax your shoulder down. Repeat with the other shoulder. Do this to a count of four up, four down. Don't move your head.

Repeat 10 times, alternating shoulders.

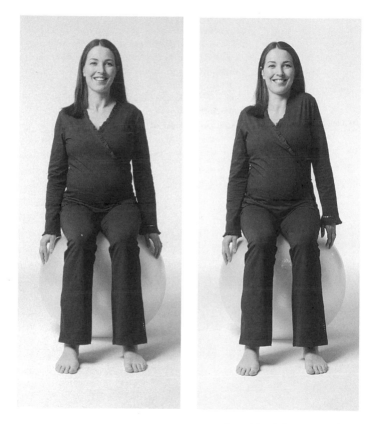

Sit comfortably on the ball with your arms relaxed at your
sides. Now queeze both shoulders up to your ears. Make
sure your hands are dangling loosely by your sides. Repeat
10 times.

Watchpoint

■ It is important not to lock your elbows or stick your neck
forward.

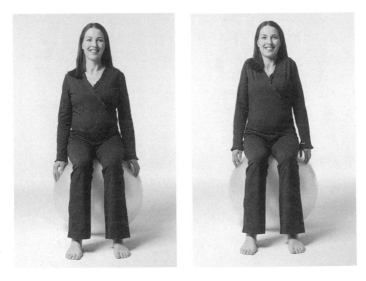

Sit comfortably on the ball with your arms relaxed at your
sides. Place your hands on your shoulders and very gently
circle both arms forward. Repeat 10 times.

Circle your arms backwards, again repeating 10 times.

If this feels uncomfortable, circle your shoulders with your
arms at your sides.

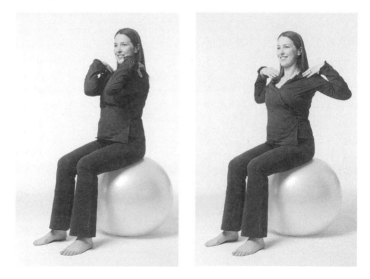

pelvic floor exercises

The reason you're working your pelvic floor muscles is that you want to keep the baby from dropping for as long as possible. You also need strong pelvic floor muscles to take the pressure off your bladder and bowel, which can cause discomfort as the baby develops and gets heavier. My clients do very minimal exercises lying on their backs after the first 14 weeks of pregnancy. There is only one included in this program, which my clients do right up to full-term.

pelvic floor exercise 1

This is like a pelvic tilt, but rather than lying down you sit on the ball, hands on your hips. Breathe in and then, very gently as you breathe out, tip your pelvic floor under. Do not pull your stomach in, but imagine the baby dropping in towards your spine.

Breathe in and arch the other way. Breathe out. Let the ball roll under you.

Repeat about 10 times.

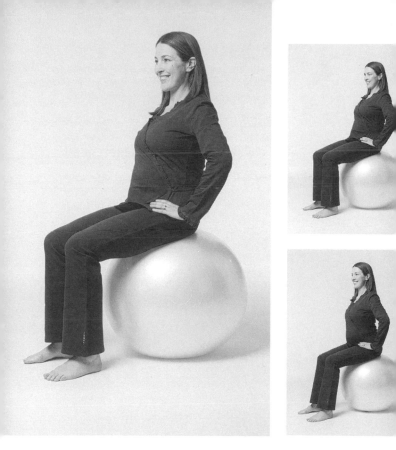

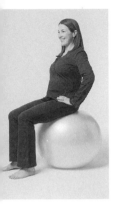

People often find these next two exercises quite difficult to start with. What you're trying to do is tighten the muscles around your pubic bone, the base of your abdominals.

Seated on the ball as in the previous exercise, breathe in, take your arms above your head, breathe out, and curl gently back. Allow the baby to drop into your spine and you will feel a tightening round the base of your pubic bone. Breathe in and sit up without arching your back. Breathe in, your arms up. Breathe out, drop back over the ball, feel the baby drop, and feel a tightening round your pubic bone.

Do approximately 10 repetitions.

It can be helpful to think of gently tightening your inner thighs as you breathe out, as this will connect with your pelvic floor muscles.

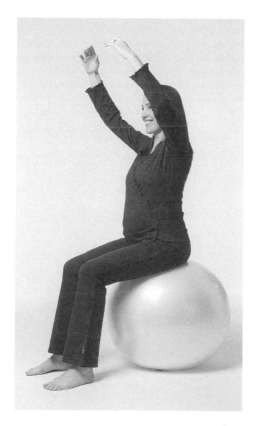

This exercise is very similar to the last one. Put your right hand around your waist. Breathe in, breathe out, think of the baby dropping back in towards your spine and raise your left arm. You will feel the muscles round your waist contracting as you lower your left arm, also the muscles round the pubic bone, the pelvic floor muscles. Breathe in and curl up.

Do 10 repetitions with alternating arms.

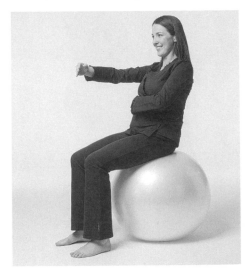

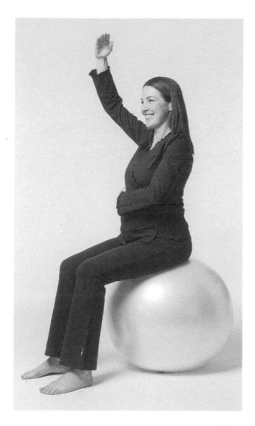

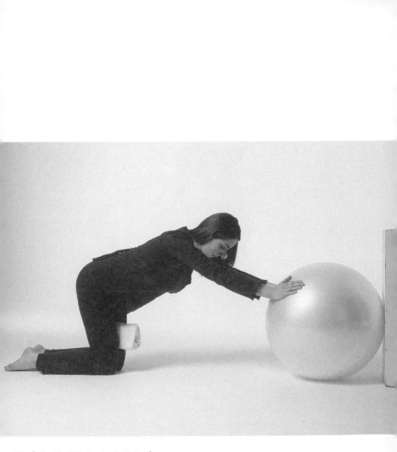

This exercise is done on your hands and knees. Have the ball supported by a wall. Kneel in a comfortable position so your hands are supported by the ball. Keep your head and neck in line, and your back flat. Your knees should be under your hips. Take a small towel between your thighs.

Breathe in, and as you breathe out squeeze the towel between your inner thighs. You will feel the base of your stomach contracting around your pelvic floor muscles. Do not allow your back to arch.

Repeat about 10 times.

Watchpoints

- It is impossible to pull your stomach in when you are pregnant. Don't think stomach – think of the deep pelvic floor muscles between the point of your anus and the point of your pubic bone.

- If you feel any discomfort in your knees, place a towel beneath them. Make sure you are securely positioned on the ball and that you feel stable before you start.

- This is an exercise you could quite easily do a second set of later in your program or later in the day.

back and thigh exercises

This is a mobilization exercise for your spine, to keep it supple.

Lie on your back with your feet on the ball, feet and legs together and tailbone on the floor. Your ankles and knees should be in line with your hips, and your feet relaxed.

Breathe in and, as you breathe out, let your legs go one way but keep your head in the center. Breathe in and bring your legs back to center. Repeat in the opposite direction. At no point move your head, nor let your shoulder blades come off the mat. Keep it a small, controlled movement. Start by doing 10 in total – that is, five to each side.

Watchpoints

- Do not let the ball take you further over than your abdominals can control the movement.

- I must stress that this is a very small movement. At no point should either shoulder blade leave the mat. Your knees should stay together as you move from side to side – this way one leg won't get longer than the other. It is very natural as you turn from side to side to take your knees further than your ankles – the movement is taken from the abdominals as your legs and the ball go from side to side.

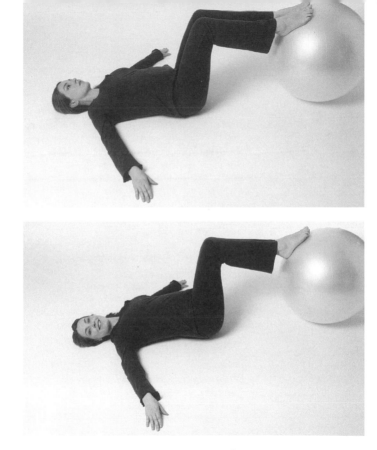

This exercise will release your lower back and stretch out your shoulders.

Support the ball against a wall. Kneel as far away as you can while still resting your palms on the ball. Keep your weight distributed evenly through to your knees. Keep your hips over your knees.

Breathe in and, as you breathe out, curl your chin into your chest and stretch out your lower back.

As you breathe in, press your chest down, your bottom up, and gently lengthen your neck.

This counts as one repetition. Repeat 10 times.

As you open your spine, this gets the blood flowing and will counteract the effects of gravity, altering your spinal integrity as the baby develops – otherwise your lower back can become overextended, which can lead to backache and, in some cases, sciatica.

Watchpoints

- If you feel your neck crunching or your vocal chords contracting, you've taken your head too far back. There should be no discomfort in your neck.

- Make sure your feet stay on the floor.

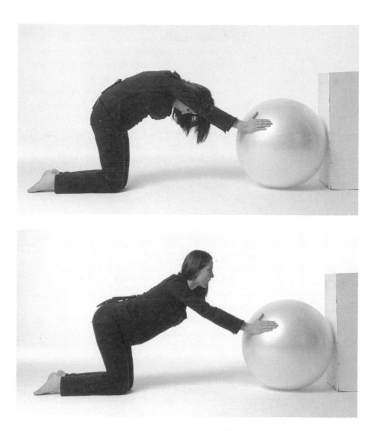

You do this one lying on your side, preferably with your back supported by a wall, and with the arm that's on the floor either supporting your head or completely flat. If you choose to keep your arm flat, it may feel more comfortable to put a towel between your arm and ear. Your other hand should be in front of you. Your top leg should be forward, in front of your body, with your foot on the ball. The underneath leg (the one that is working) needs to be slightly forward, with your foot gently flexed. Don't lock your knee, but pull up the muscles so that your leg is straight. If your legs are not straight, you'll be working your ankle and your foot much more than your inside thigh.

Lie on your left side and breathe in. As you breathe out, lift your left leg and hold. As you lift and breathe out, feel your waist toning as well as your inner thigh. The energy is through your heel, working your inner thigh. Do 10 with your left leg, then turn onto your right side and do 10 with your right leg.

Watchpoints

■ It is important for this exercise, particularly after the fifth month of pregnancy, that you lie with your back against a wall so that both hips are supported by it and there is no strain in your lumbar spine. It will probably be more comfortable for you with your head on your arm.

■ Make sure your hips are in line, "stacked" one on top of the other.

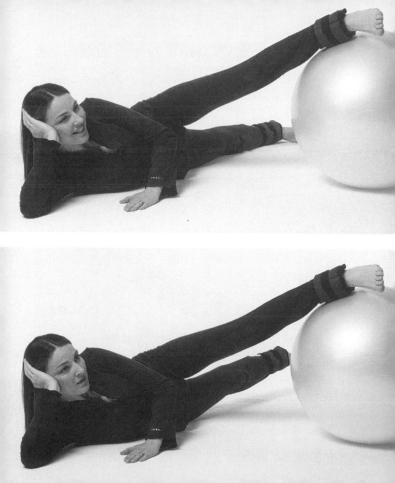

Lie on your left side, as in the previous exercise. Lift your
left leg, bend your knee gently, and "squeeze" to straighten
your leg. Keep your foot gently flexed and your knee
unlocked. You may want to place a small towel between
your arm and your ear for comfort.

Repeat 10 times, keeping your leg in the air the whole time
as you bend it. Do 10 on the other side.

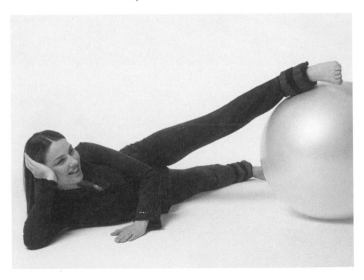

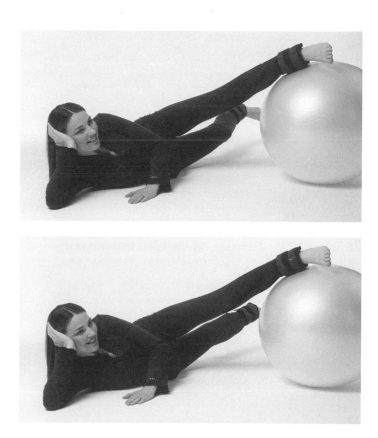

upper body exercises

Now you're ready to continue with your upper body toning
and strengthening. Kneel down with your hands on the floor
in front of the ball, your feet behind the ball.

Carefully walk forwards until your hips are on the ball and
your feet are off the floor. Only go as far over the ball as
feels comfortable. Your hands are under your shoulders –
just wider than shoulder-width apart, with the palms flat
and fingers pointing away from you. Keeping your head in
line, gently tip your weight forwards.

Breathe in as you bend your arms, breathe out as you
straighten them, keeping your back stable. Repeat 10 times.

Watchpoints

- The further over the ball you are, the less stable you are and
  the harder you have to work.

- Keep your legs together and your inside thighs gently
  squeezed to feel more stable.

- It's very important not to arch your back. The alignment of
  your neck and upper back is essential.

- Try not to seesaw or let your legs go up and down.

- As well as toning arms and upper back, this is essential for core stability.

- This is an exercise you must use your judgement on. Some of my clients carry on doing this up until quite late stages of pregnancy, some do not. Slightly later on in the program you will see an alternative press-up against a wall. If you have any discomfort around where the baby is lying, do the alternative press-ups *(see page 382)*.

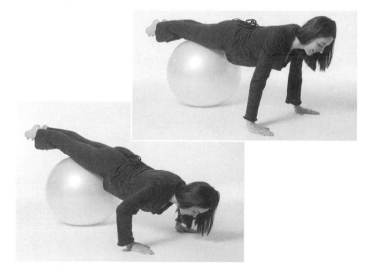

Make sure the ball is secured by a wall. Place your left
hand on the ball and kneel behind it, keeping your right arm
straight to the ground. Keep your neck in line with the rest
of your body. Holding a hand weight (a can of beans or
bottle of water will do), inhale and lift your right elbow up as
high as you can, keeping your elbow bent at a right angle,
without twisting your body. Exhale as you straighten your

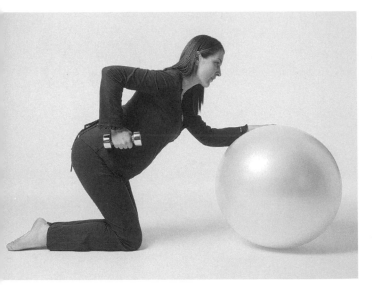

arm behind you. Pause. Bend your arm back again. Hold
the ball and lean as far over the ball as you feel secure.

Repeat 10–15 times on each arm – this is one "set". You
may do a second set.

Watchpoint

- At no point allow your back to arch.

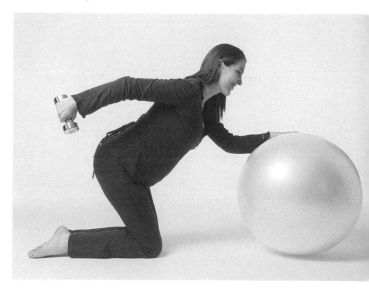

Sit on the ball with a two-kilo/four-pound weight in each hand. Breathe in and bend your arm up to shoulder level. Breathe out and straighten to waist level. Try not to rock as you do this. Repeat 10 to 15 times with alternate arms.

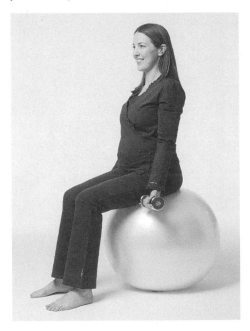

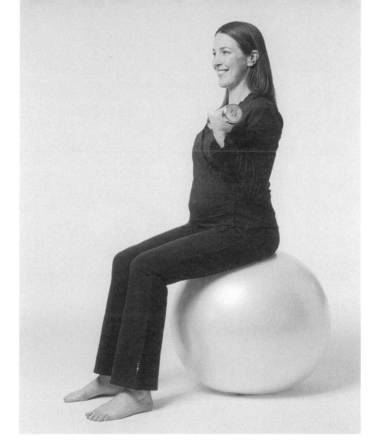

standing calf stretch

Stand up straight, holding the ball in your hands against a wall. Take a step forward with your left leg and, leaning against the ball, bend your knee slightly and feel the stretch down through your right leg. Keep your right heel down. Do not bounce. Hold for 30 seconds. Repeat four times, alternating legs.

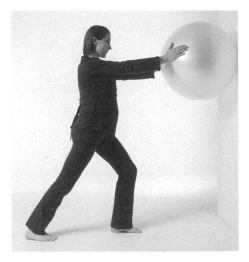

Kneel down on your right leg, keeping your back straight,
and rest your hands on the ball, which should be
supported against a solid surface. Then extend your left
leg straight, making sure that your heel is always in front
of your knee. Gently relax the baby into your spine and
lean back slightly, making sure you don't arch your back.
Hold for 30 seconds.

Repeat twice for each leg.

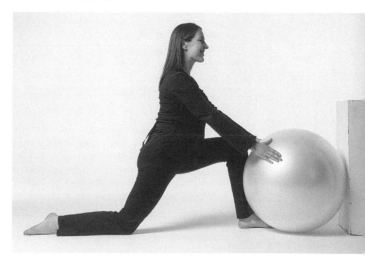

This is one of only two exercises not on the ball, as using the ball would be too unstable.

Seated on a chair, starting with both feet on the ground, raise and cross your right ankle over your left knee. Breathe in, then very gently breathe out and lean forward. Try to lean over your bent (right) knee and you will feel a stretch in the back of your hip and buttock. Keep your head, neck, and shoulders relaxed. Hold for 20 seconds.

Gently press your right knee down, without either pulling on your ankle and foot or twisting your pelvis. If this feels uncomfortable, you can always put your left foot on a telephone directory to lift it slightly higher.

Repeat four times on each leg, alternating legs.

Watchpoint

■ It is absolutely vital to stretch out the back of the hip muscles when you are pregnant, due to the fact that gravity is constantly creating an overarched lumbar spine, which can cause lumbar and back problems and sciatica. Basically, my pregnant clients don't get sciatica because we do a huge amount of mobilization and strengthening to avoid a strain in the lumbar spine. This can be caused by the change in posture, the problems with gravity as the body changes, and the weight of the baby constantly tipping you forward.

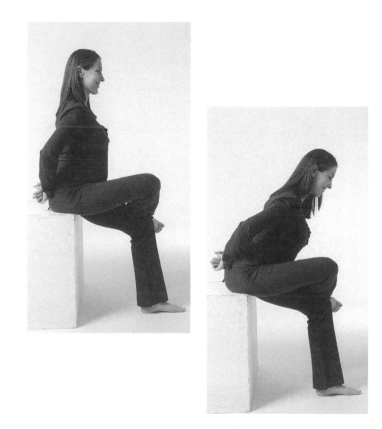

BUTTOCK TONING

Many of my clients do the earlier buttock-toning exercises over the ball *(see pages 315–317)* up to the point where they no longer feel comfortable on the ball. Again, you can use your judgement during your earlier stages of pregnancy.

stronger stretches

This exercise will stretch the back of your legs. You must make sure that whatever you are using to support your leg is a very stable surface. The height of the box or whatever you use is relevant to how tight your legs are. This varies from person to person. And as you get bigger, you may need to change the height, possibly taking it lower.

Place your right foot, gently flexed, on a stable surface and extend your leg. Keep your left leg slightly bent and your neck and shoulders relaxed. Hips are level. Slide your hands down towards your right foot. You should feel the stretch in the muscle between your knee and the hip. Hold for 20 seconds. Repeat four times, alternating legs.

Watchpoints

- Keep the leg you are standing on slightly bent.

- It is really important when you are pregnant that you don't do developmental stretching, because the ligaments and the tendons soften to allow for the birth of the baby. A lot of people get confused and think that they are actually more flexible. This is not true. If you overstretch a tendon or ligament during pregnancy, it will remain overstretched after the birth. The female body is perfectly designed for everything to return to normal after giving birth, but obviously not if you have overstretched.

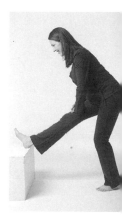

Place the ball against a wall, with your palms as wide as
possible on the ball slightly below shoulder level. Breathe
in as you bend your elbows and come towards the ball;
breathe out as you straighten.

Repeat about 10 times – but as this is less demanding
than press-ups over the ball, do an extra set when you feel
comfortable with the exercise.

Watchpoints

■ Keep your neck and shoulders in line.

■ Do not arch your lower back.

■ You will know if you are too far away from the ball, as your
   heels will leave the ground.

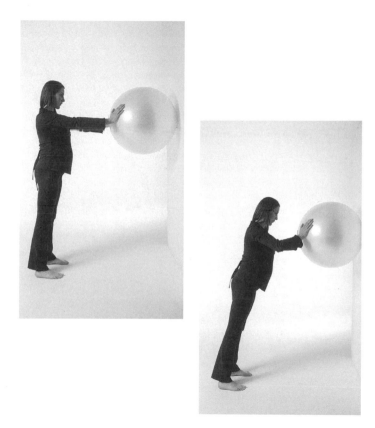

For this first shoulder stretch, you are kneeling down. Your bottom is resting on your heels. If you feel you have very tight feet and/or your feet are uncomfortable, you can put a towel under them.

Place the palm of your right hand on the center of the ball. As you breathe out, push the ball as far as it will go without lifting your bottom. Breathe in and come back to an upright position. As you breathe out feel your shoulder stretching, the shoulder blade gliding up towards your ear, then relaxing back as you breathe in.

Let your head and neck just flow along your arm in a relaxed, soft movement. If your neck feels uncomfortable you are probably in the wrong position, so adjust it until your neck feels comfortable. Your elbow should not be locked at any point.

Do 10 repetitions on each arm.

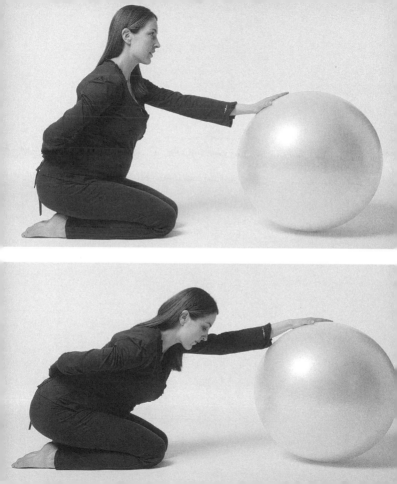

This exercise is much more challenging. Start in the same position as for the Single Shoulder Stretch, but place both hands on the sides of the ball. Breathe in, then as you breathe out push the ball away from you, pushing your chest to the floor as your bottom comes off your heels. Breathe in and come back.

Watchpoints

- Keep your ears between your arms the whole time. Most people drop their head too low. It's just as important not to lift your head too high so you feel a pinching in your neck.

- Do not let your feet leave the ground.

- This is an upper body stretch, so if you feel any discomfort in your lower back, you are working incorrectly and pushing the ball too far away.

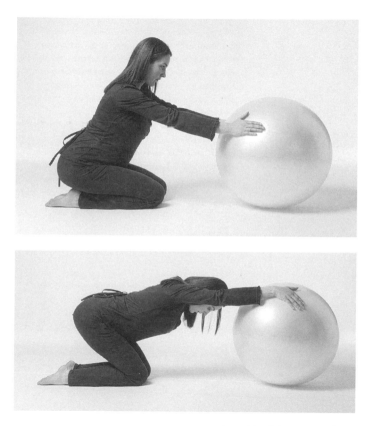

This is the alternative to the previous kneeling exercise, and is useful for anyone with either bad knees or a serious lumbar condition. It is exactly the same exercise except that you push the ball up a wall. Many of my pregnant clients replace the kneeling shoulder stretch with this standing wall stretch as their pregnancy develops.

Stand with complete Pilates postural integrity, feet hip-width apart, tailbone dropped, head and neck in line, ears between your raised arms, elbows released. Breathe in and, as you breathe out, push the ball up the wall *(see page 390)*. Do not lock your elbows, do not arch your back. Make sure the ball is against a secure surface.

Repeat 10 times.

Watchpoint
- If you are too far away from the wall your heels will come off the ground and your back will arch. If you are too close you will not get any stretch.

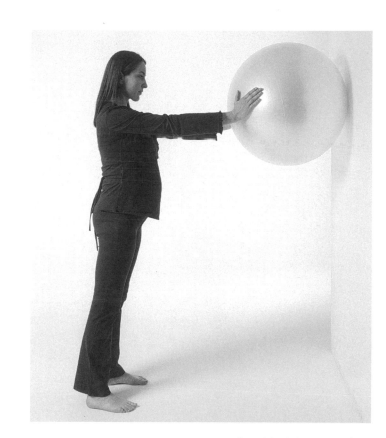

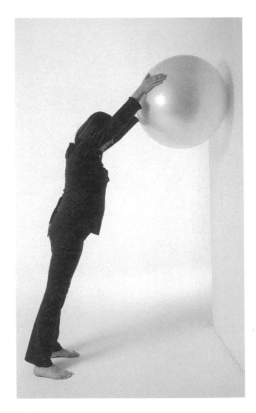

ONE MOTHER'S STORY

Julia Daly started taking Lesley's classes to help with her recurring lower back pain, then discovered how it helped her through her second pregnancy.

"I started seeing Lesley about seven months after the birth of my first son, Louis. My lower back would go into spasms and I wouldn't be able to move for three, sometimes five days. I'd have to take a lot of painkillers and be carried in to see an osteopath. I was worried about the pain getting worse with a child in tow. Although I was sceptical that Pilates could help with such chronic pain, I have not had to visit the osteopath once since I started my sessions, twice a week, in 1999.

When I got pregnant again Lesley devised a suitable program for me. We concentrated on the pelvic floor and some very gentle stomach exercises. These were done by lifting the stomach towards the spine, flattening it rather than contracting the stomach muscles. About 13 weeks into my pregnancy Lesley stopped me from doing any exercises on my back because the weight of the baby would put pressure on major veins. I continued with all the arm and leg exercises, and some modified waist exercises, using the Physio Ball. Lesley tailored the program to my body type as well: because I have long legs and a relatively short back, she would make sure I wouldn't lift my legs too high, for example. She always erred on the side of caution and made sure I didn't overextend myself. As the sessions were strengthening but nonetheless fairly gentle, I was showing up regularly right up until I started getting contractions. Lesley sent me home even though I was prepared to stay and finish the class! Two days later I gave birth to my second son, Freddie.

My second pregnancy was much easier because of Pilates. As it's a lengthening program, I felt that I had room in my body for my baby. Some pregnant women can't eat full meals towards the end of their pregnancy, but I never felt like my body was being overtaken by this child. By strengthening my spine and maintaining my posture through Pilates I was able to resist another common problem of the back arching inwards, which also causes terrible back pains.

During my first pregnancy I often felt I was tuned in to eight radio stations at once, with my mind constantly worrying about so many things at the same time. Attending two 90-minute classes a week during my second pregnancy really helped me take my mind off everything else and focus on just one thing, because the exercises require so much concentration, which was also very relaxing. I would come into each session after I'd been rushing around and I would leave feeling very at peace with myself.

Although I don't work up a sweat as I would in an aerobics class, I always feel I've worked out after Pilates. As a low-impact strengthening program it definitely helped when it came to labor, as I felt I could ride the exhaustion out more easily. If you stop breastfeeding quite soon then you can go back to exercising on a more rigorous basis, but I did it gradually, and six months after Freddie was born I was completely back to normal. Despite carrying two heavy boys all the time, my back has never felt stronger. I don't have the aches and pains of my friends who have children.

Many pregnant women don't get their waistline back, but with Pilates my waist is better than it has ever been. I really like the body shape Pilates has given me. It has broadened my shoulder line, nipped in my waist, and really lengthened me. Lesley's arm exercises have also prevented my bust from travelling south! I'm toned but it doesn't look 'worked', and that's all due to the Pilates. People think I've lost weight, even though I haven't. It's like I've redistributed the weight in a nicer fashion."

The benefits of embarking on a Pilates-based exercise program are manifold. As in any DIY book, until you familiarize yourself with all the material and go through it at your own pace, it may seem a bit confusing. You will find that once you coordinate your movements with the correct breathing any apprehension will soon vanish.

conclusion

While the material is still fresh, before you close this book, why not try some of the simple visualization exercises right now? Close your eyes and scan your body, visiting each area. What do you feel? Is any area painful or weak? Do you immediately focus on one area? Try some of the simple postural exercises to get a feeling of alignment. Imagine how you wish to appear.

Your body represents the sum of its parts – therefore each part must be fully conversant with the others. Fluency can be achieved by allowing the mind–body–spirit connection to evolve. This is a challenge that can be met with calm determination and a vision of purpose.

Everybody's potential is limitless. We can look forward to aging well, living longer, and having more productive lives. We often pay no attention to our bodies until something goes wrong. The human body is a splendid vehicle. Like a car, it requires regular maintenance, especially since it can't be traded in. Our bodies remain with us all our lives. It is not costly or painful to respect and maintain them.

With Pilates you can slowly re-create a sense of physical vitality and core stability, and look forward to continued wellbeing and health. You now have the tools. Good luck!

index

H

hamstrings 54
   lying stretch 144–5, 324–5
   standing stretch 142–3, 381
   toner/strengthener 122, 318–19
hands
   program 212–13
   stretch 240
healthcare professionals 342–3
height 67–8
Herdman, Alan 21
hips
   basic stretch 228–9, 234
   flexor 150–1
   gluteal stretch 128–31, 321
   mobility 180–3
   rolls 226–7, 310–11, 362–3
HIV-related problems 21
hyperextension 50

I

imbalances 18, 346
inner thighs 266–9
   advanced stretch 148–9
   circles 116
   lift 114–15, 312–14
   stretch 146–7
intercellular communication 27
internal oblique 56
inversion 52
Ireland, Jane 345–7

J

jewelry 60

K

key terms 47–9
kneeling arm/leg stretch 106–7, 304–5

L

lat exercise 162–3
latissimus dorsi 56
leg lifts, straight 292–5
leg stretches 126–51
   alternate 104–5
   kneeling 106–7, 304–5
   toning 312–25
legs 48–9
   program 376–80
   straight 48–9
   strengthening 112–25
levator scapulae 54
lower abdominals 286–9, 296–7
   program 81–3
lower back, passive stretch 224
lying exercises
   calf stretch 138–9
   hamstring stretch 144–5, 324–5

M

mat work 24, 60
media 16, 342–3, 344
midday break 204–17
mind over matter 27–8
mindfulness 30–1
mirrors 62
miscarriage 343
mobilization 175, 264
morning energizer 175–7
movements 50–2
muscles 52–6

N

natural fibers 60
neck 49, 64
   stretch 202–3
neutral spine 47